I just wanted to say thanks for publishing such a great cookbook. I was diagnosed with Candida in January and being a very bad cook myself, I had no idea how I was going to work through the yeast free diet. I have cooked several of the recipes in your book now and my husband and I both enjoyed them very much.

Thanks again,
Susan Smith

I am writing to thank you for your excellent book *The Candida Control Cookbook*. I have been testing your recipes for me and my family for the last week. We had been eating such bland and boring food on my candida diet and your recipes and information have helped us find food that we enjoy. We especially like the Festive Pumpkin and Nut Muffins and the Chicken Cutlets Italiano. I can not wait to taste more. I am sorry that you suffered with candida but please know that you are making life better for others like me. I appreciate you so very much.

May God bless you in all things.
Debbie Ross

I want to thank you and to tell you about my success story. I truly believe that my body constantly deals with candida yeast infection. I would imagine that I've had it a long time. I feel like I have my life back. I'm now in control. It would not have happened if I had not bought your book I've been overweight for 20 years. Because of your book, I've lost 55 lbs.! I follow the candida control diet and use your recipes. I believe that I will follow this diet for the rest of my life. I've actually grown accustomed to it and like it! I also powerwalk and run. I find that its very meditative.

I feel like telling the entire world about your *Candida Control Cookbook!* I too believe that many people have this infection and have no idea. Thanks again! I hope you feel my excitement. You have done a wonderful thing with this book.

Bette Wappner

CANDIDA
THE SILENT EPIDEMIC

Gail Burton is also the author of

The Candida Control Cookbook

What You Should Know
and What You Should Eat
to Manage Yeast Infections

CANDIDA
THE SILENT EPIDEMIC

SECOND EDITION

Vital Information to
Detect, Combat, and *Prevent*
Yeast Infections

GAIL BURTON

With an Introduction by
Michael E. Rosenbaum, M.D.

Foreword by
Michael M. McNett, M.D.

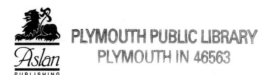

Disclaimer
The information contained in this book is not intended as medical advice.
It is recommended that the reader consult a health care professional for any
medical condition. The publishers and author expressly disclaim any liability for
injuries resulting from use by readers of the methods contained herein.

Library of Congress Cataloging-in-Publication Data

Burton, Gail
    Candida : the silent epidemic : vital information to detect, combat,
and prevent yeast infections / Gail Burton ; with an introduction by
Michael E. Rosenbaum, ; foreword by Michael M. McNett.
        p. cm.
    Previously published: Woodbury, Minn. : G. Burton, 1999.
    Includes bibliographical references and index.
    ISBN 0-944031-93-5 (alk. paper)
        1. Candidiasis—Popular works. I. Title.

RC123.C3B873 2003
616.9′69—dc21   2003051853

Published by:
Aslan Publishing
2490 Black Rock Turnpike #342
Fairfield, CT 06825
Order line: 800-786-5427
www.aslanpublishing.com

Printed in the United States of America

This book is dedicated
to the memory of
Keith W. Sehnert, M.D.
who inspired me with his great
knowledge, enthusiasm, and courage
to help others recover from Candida
and Candida-related complex (CRC).

CONTENTS

Contents

Contents

ACKNOWLEDGMENTS

Michael E. Rosenbaum, M.D., Corte Madera, CA, for diagnosing and successfully treating me for chronic Candidiasis. Also, for writing this book's Introduction.

Michael M. McNett, M.D., owner/medical director, Paragon Clinic, Chicago, IL, for referring my books to many patients who suffer with *Candida,* fibromyalgia, chronic muscular pain, and Myofascial Pain Syndrome. Also, for writing this book's Foreword.

Adiel Tel-Oren, D.C., M.D., CCN, DABCN, FABDA, founder/ director of Integrated HealthCare Clinics, Inc., Minneapolis, MN, for suggesting this book's title and for his valuable information in the chapter, "Why *Candida* Sufferers May Not Recover."

Leo B. Cashman, Minneapolis health writer, for providing vital information in the section, "The Removal of Silver Amalgams," as well as the chapter, "Protecting Your Rights to Safe, Alternative Health Care."

Barbara and Harold Levine, for publishing *The Candida Control Cookbook*, as well as this book. Also, for Barbara's wonderful book, *Your Body Believes Every Word You Say: The Language of the Body/Mind Connection, 2nd ed.*

Allen S. Weiss, *Candida* recoverer and special friend, for his generous help and ideas.

Holly LeGros, for information on MCS (Multiple Chemical Sensitivities) and other help.

Catherine Thornton, for her kind help and information.

Sheila Ambrose, for her expertise and ideas.

All sufferers who made me realize the necessity for this book to assist in detecting, combating, and preventing *Candida.*

ABOUT THE AUTHOR

Gail Burton, a food columnist and employee counselor, suffered with misdiagnosed illness for over 10 years. In 1985, Dr. Michael Rosenbaum, of Corte Madera, California, finally correctly diagnosed her with chronic Candidiasis, yeast infection.

Dr. Rosenbaum put her on the *Candida* Treatment Program, but it was difficult for her to stay on the *Candida* Control Diet because it was so restrictive. However, she realized that the special diet helped her symptoms and that, to be able to stay on it, she needed to have enjoyable recipes. She did a great deal of experimentation to create meals and desserts with good substitutions for problem ingredients.

Her results were so successful that Dr. Rosenbaum asked her to write a cookbook for other *Candida* sufferers. When she learned that millions of people all over the world were infected with *Candida* and that a good cookbook was badly needed, she immediately went to work. After more than two years of research on *Candida* and as much recipe testing, she wrote *The Candida Control Cookbook: What You Should Know and What You Should Eat to Manage Yeast Infections*. Published since 1989 and updated many times, it is considered to be the best cookbook on the market for *Candida* control.

Gail felt so fortunate to recover that she wanted to help many others. She was a counselor at the former *Candida* Research and Information Foundation, and she has been a director/counselor for *Candida* support groups with hundreds of members, in both California and Minnesota. She has done a great deal of individual counseling, and has been featured on national television and radio several times.

It still concerned her that so many people who were infected with *Candida* couldn't make full recovery. She did further research to find the answers, which are in this book.

Readers should greatly benefit from the author's expertise in research and in relaying what she has learned.

FOREWORD
by Michael M. McNett, M.D.

For most conditions, medical care is pretty straightforward. A person goes to a doctor with a specific complaint, the history, exam, and lab tests point to a likely cause, and effective treatment is provided.

For many people, however, this system doesn't seem to work. They suffer from a variety of vague but disturbing problems such as fatigue, diffuse pain, recurring infections, allergies, ineffective sleep, intestinal problems, irritable bladder, emotional upheavals, or difficulty concentrating. These and many other problems may come and go without apparent cause, disrupting their life and causing them misery. They go from doctor to doctor, get innumerable tests (all of which come back normal), and are told, "We can't find anything wrong. It's all in your head—you're too stressed."

Of course they're stressed. They're stressed because they're miserable. They can't figure out what's happening to them, and medical science doesn't seem able to help them. They're stressed because they're sick, not the other way around.

There may, however, be hope. A few visionary doctors had the insight to realize that these symptoms might be caused by a yeast (*Candida*) overgrowth in the intestines. This awareness started with J.A. Buchanan, M.D., in 1923 with his article, "Significance of Yeast in Stomach and Intestines," and was developed in the 1980s by C. Orion Truss, M.D., in *The Missing Diagnosis* and William Crook, M.D., in *The Yeast Connection*. Unfortunately, there were no good scientific studies confirming the existence of the condition. As a result, most physicians remained unconvinced of its validity and refused to treat it.

Recently, however, a well-done study has clearly shown the

xiii

benefit of treating *Candida* overgrowth, as described in "Effectiveness of Nystatin in Polysymptomatic Patients," by H. Santelmann, E. Laerum, J. Ronnevig, and H.E. Fagertun (*Family Practice Journal* 2001).

Hopefully, physicians will now become more aware of the condition and provide patients the help they so desperately need.

Gail Burton has done *Candida* sufferers a great favor with this book. In a precise and succinct way, she has summarized the main causes, symptoms, and treatments for *Candida* overgrowth. Specific dietary and lifestyle guidelines are provided that can go a long way toward relieving the *Candida* patient's suffering. Having been a *Candida* patient herself, she brings a tremendous understanding of the condition to her writing and guides the readers to the answers they seek.

If you have multiple, unexplained medical problems, this book may help you find your answers. I recommend it wholeheartedly.

Michael M. McNett, M.D.

NOTE: Dr. McNett specializes in fibromyalgia and muscular pain. He is owner and medical director of Paragon Clinic.
Address: 4332 N. Elston Ave., Chicago, IL 60641
Phone: 773-604-5321.
Website: www.paragonclinic.com
E-mail: mmcnett@paragonclinic.com

PREFACE

Candida, the Silent Epidemic is just that! I say that *Candida* is silent because most people aren't aware they have *Candida*—yeast infection—which is frequently misdiagnosed.

Misdiagnosis occurs because many traditional physicians aren't familiar with *Candida.* They didn't study it in medical school. Also, they can misdiagnose because *Candida* symptoms are typical of many other conditions. In addition, they often consider those patients to be hypochondriacs due to complaints of vast and diverse symptoms—or they believe that depression is causing the problems.

Candida is an epidemic, because it has infected millions of people all over the world. It is widespread because of our "modern-day miracle drugs": antibiotics, steroids, anti-inflammatory and pain medications, antidepressants, hormones, and birth-control pills. Chemicals, molds, stress, too much sugar in our diets, and many other factors can cause *Candida.*

I am referring not only to ordinary vaginal yeast infections, but also to systemic *Candidiasis,* which can cause many problems internally. The problems result from toxins from the *Candida albicans* yeast, which can affect the body from the brain all the way to the colon.

I have counseled many *Candida* sufferers all over the world. Some people were so ill that they could hardly work, while others could barely function. Many had other conditions along with *Candida,* which are referred to as *Candida*-Related Complex (CRC): lupus, chronic fatigue syndrome, multiple sclerosis, rheumatoid arthritis, fibromyalgia, leaky gut syndrome, allergies, thyroid and/or adrenal dysfunction, spastic colon, parasites, and much more.

It bothered me that so many people could get infected with *Candida,* but couldn't make full recovery. I wanted to find out why this was happening. After a great deal of research, I found many answers to this puzzle.

I wanted to inform *Candida* sufferers of what I had learned, so I wrote this self-help book. It contains significant information to help readers to self-evaluate whether they may have *Candida.* The book also has answers to the question of why many people who receive treatment are not able to recover. In addition, there is vital information on how sufferers may regain their health. Finally, for individuals who haven't yet been infected, there is helpful information on how to prevent *Candida.*

I know that, when you read this book, you will learn new and valuable information that will enable you to obtain and maintain good health.

Best wishes,
Gail Burton

INTRODUCTION
by Michael E. Rosenbaum, M.D.

It is a privilege for me to write the Introduction to Gail Burton's new book, *Candida: The Silent Epidemic*. This is an excellent companion edition to Gail's first book, *The Candida Control Cookbook*, which has over the past decade achieved much success and recognition as a popular dietary guide to living with yeast-related illnesses.

Gail Burton has first-hand knowledge of "*Candida*-Related Complex" (CRC). She endured 10 years of debilitating pain and inflammation, which was largely eradicated in 1985 by a strict food allergy and antiyeast regimen. She has dedicated much of her subsequent efforts to educating other patients about the causes, treatment, and prevention of yeast-related illnesses. Indeed, in this compact book she details the extent of the yeast problem in modern society and its numerous potential causes:

- widespread use of antibiotics in pill form and hidden in meat and poultry
- a diet high in sweets and high-glycemic foods
- use of steroid drugs
- exposure to toxic chemicals and heavy metals
- chronic stress

Having practiced nutritional medicine with a focus on nutrition and immunity for the past 25 years, I know the harmful effects of stress, sweets, steroids, and toxic chemicals on the immune response. *Candida* is an opportunistic organism that multiplies when immune reserves are low and in its aggressive mycelial form it secretes endotoxins that may elicit a pro-inflammatory response.

Gail does not just present the problems, she furnishes questionnaires and symptom lists to help readers assess their own potential for yeast-related complaints. She also furnishes numerous practical dietary solutions to help patients deal more effectively with their treatment. What impressed me was her style of delivering comprehensive information with plain talk—simple, to the point, and easy to understand. She tells you what to eat and how to shop, and provides a list of valuable resources for contacting organizations in this field. I highly recommend this book as an invaluable adjunct to a medically supervised yeast management program.

Michael E. Rosenbaum, M.D.

NOTE: Dr. Rosenbaum specializes in Nutrition, Allergy, Immunology and Anti-aging.
Address: 300 Tamal Plaza, Suite 120,
Corte Madera, CA 94925.
Phone: 414-927-9450
Website: www.michaelrosenbaummd.com
E-mail: mermd@michaelrosenbaummd.com

I. What is *Candida*?

Candida or *Candidiasis* is a yeast infection. It can also become a fungal infection.

The word *Candida* comes from the *Candida albicans* yeast, which commonly grow in our mucous membranes, intestines, vagina, and on the skin. The yeast are usually harmless, unless certain factors cause them to become active, multiply, and release toxins, which then produce symptoms from head to toe.

Systemic *Candidiasis* can affect a person internally from the brain, to the ears, nose, sinuses, mouth, intestinal tract and colon, the upper respiratory, cardiovascular and pulmonary systems, the adrenal and thyroid glands, the muscles and joints, the urinary tract, vaginal, and anal areas. *Candida* can also affect the skin.

Candida has even been known to cause allergic reactions, as well as malabsorption of valuable nutrients. Some people may have mild infections of *Candida*. Others may be so ill with (CC) Chronic *Candidiasis* or Systemic *Candidiasis* that they can hardly work. Still others can barely function.

Candida-Related Complex (CRC)

When other health conditions become involved, *Candida* becomes known as *Candida*-Related Complex (CRC). This can include Chronic Fatigue Syndrome, Hypoglycemia, Leaky Gut Syndrome, Fibromyalgia, allergy or sensitivity, hormonal, thyroid, and adrenal dysfunction, emotion-related disorders, and many more conditions.

The book, *CANDIDA-RELATED COMPLEX: What Your Doctor Might Be Missing*, by Christin Winderlin with Keith Sehnert, M.D., describes CRC in great detail.

Traditional Doctors and *Candida*

Many traditional doctors do not recognize *Candida* because they didn't study it in medical school. They were taught how to pre-scribe medications like antibiotics, steroids, pain and anti-in-flammatory drugs, diuretics, antidepressants, hormones, birth-control pills, and so on, all of which can cause *Candida*.

When a patient comes to a physician with complaints of many symptoms, as is typical of *Candida*, many times the pa-tient is either considered to be a hypochondriac or depressed. As a result, many people have been misdiagnosed.

Today, more and more physicians and health care practition-ers are becoming aware of *Candida* and are treating patients for the condition. (See the Foreword by Michael E. McNett, M.D.)

The state of Minnesota was usually very conservative when it came to alternative health care. However, it has taken great steps in recognizing alternative medicine. The University of Minnesota opened its first Alternative Medicine Clinic at Fairview University Medical Center in Minneapolis during the summer of 1999, and the university was the first in the country to teach Alternative Medicine in its graduate program, which began in fall 1999.

Today, many other states are acknowledging alternative medicine. It is important to be open to alternatives to success-fully treat *Candida*.

Please see Chapter VIII, "Protecting Your Rights to Safe, Al-ternative Health care," by Leo B. Cashman, Minneapolis health writer.

Who Can Be Infected with *Candida*?

Anyone can be infected with *Candida* today! Women can be infected because of antibiotics, steroids, pain and anti-inflammatory medications, hormones and birth-control pills, sexual relations with an infected partner, and many other factors. (See Chapter II, "*Candida*-Causing Factors.")

Men can also be infected with *Candida* from antibiotics, steroids, anti-inflammatory drugs, pain medications, sexual relations with an infected partner, and many more factors.

Teenagers get *Candida* from routine treatment with tetracycline or other antibiotics for acne. As a result, they may have many symptoms, especially depression, because of the toxins from *Candida,* which can affect the brain. As a result, some teenagers have even become suicidal.

Children can easily get *Candida* from being treated with antibiotics for ear infections. When antibiotics kill the bad bacteria, the good bacteria are affected as well. When this happens, a child may become predisposed to getting recurring ear infections. So it becomes a vicious cycle: ear infection—antibiotics— ear infection—antibiotics—ear infection, and so on.

When babies have *Candida*, they've usually gotten it from the birth canal or breast milk of the infected mother. That is why babies often have thrush (a white-coated tongue), which is yeast infection.

Millions of people all over the world are infected with *Candida*. At least one out of three people in the Western world are affected. Because so many of our population can be infected and because so many factors can cause the condition, *Candida* is an enormous health problem today.

II. *Candida*-Causing Factors

Many factors can cause *Candida* overgrowth, including . . .

* medications
* invasive procedures
* diseases and autoimmune diseases
* chemicals
* molds
* mercury in silver amalgam dental fillings
* parasites
* too much sugar/complex carbohydrates
* stress

The following sections tell you more about each of these.

Medications

Prescription drugs taken for a long time—or repeatedly—can cause *Candida*. Antibiotics, especially, can cause *Candida,* as can steroids like cortisone and prednisone. Also, pain medications, anti-inflammatory drugs, antidepressants, diuretics, anticoagulants, estrogen and progesterone, and birth-control pills can cause *Candida.*

Those medications and others can eradicate the good bacteria along with the bad. When a person doesn't have the bacteria necessary to fight viruses, infections, and disease, more health problems can readily occur.

If one's diet regularly includes meat and poultry grown on most domestic farms in this country, antibiotics and steroids are also consumed because they are routinely fed to the animals. This produces unwanted and undesirable results for humans. The use of organically grown meat products is preferred. If a person cannot afford the more-expensive natural meats and poultry during treatment, it is preferable to eat vegetarian foods—such as vegetables and grains without wheat-containing gluten.

Invasive Procedures

Often, invasive procedures like surgery, implants, radiation, and chemotherapy can cause *Candida,* because the immune system becomes impaired. When the immune system is weakened, the *Candida albicans* yeast, which are normally harmless, become active, multiply, and can cause symptoms from head to toe.

Diseases and Autoimmune Disorders

Diseases and autoimmune disorders can indirectly cause *Candida*, by causing the immune system to become deficient. When this happens, the normally harmless *Candida albicans* yeast living in the mucous membranes, intestinal tract, and vagina, can become active and harmful.

An autoimmune disorder develops when there are cells and/or antibodies arising from and directed against the individual's own tissue. Autoimmune disorders include: lupus, multiple sclerosis, rheumatoid arthritis, Crohn's disease, HIV infection, scleroderma, thyroiditis, Graves' disease, myasthenia gravis, hepatitis, and others.

Many times, *Candida* symptoms may actually be worse than the symptoms from the primary disease or autoimmune disorder. That is because the *Candida albicans* produce toxins that can affect the brain, mouth, esophagus, intestinal tract, and colon. The toxins can also affect the cardiovascular system, adrenal and thyroid glands, as well as the skin. For example, AIDS patients have been known to suffer more with thrush (yeast infection) of the mouth, throat, and esophagus than from other aspects of their disease.

Also, treatments for disease and/or autoimmune disorders, such as antibiotics, steroids, and other medications, can cause yeast overgrowth and destroy the necessary good bacteria that prevent yeast overgrowth. It is therefore necessary to control the yeast, to reduce their toxins and take pressure off of the immune system.

Many individuals who suffer from diseases or autoimmune disorders have shown significant improvement after receiving antiyeast/antifungal treatment and observing the *Candida* Control Diet.

Chemicals

People who are subjected to chemicals in their home or workplace can become very ill. The toxins from the chemicals and the toxins stimulated by *Candida* can attack the immune system, causing all kinds of harmful effects.

Many times individuals have construction, painting, or cleaning done in their home while they live in it. They may not be aware that they could become quite ill from the chemicals used in those processes.

There are many harmful chemicals used routinely in the home for cleaning. There have also been reports of wood or linoleum flooring with harmful chemicals in their sealing process, or damaging chemicals in rug padding. If a person has sensitivity to chemicals, use of natural cleaning and painting products is recommended.

Natural cleaning products are often available in natural foods stores and co-ops, as well as from companies that specialize in them. They can be found in the yellow pages.

Many people who have *Candida* have also been affected by multichemical sensitivity (MCS). MCS has been known to affect the immune system, which enables the *Candida albicans* yeast to become active, multiply, and flourish. Once this happens, the toxins from the *Candida,* as well as those from the chemicals, can wreak havoc throughout the body. (See "Holly Suffered from *Candida* and MCS," in Chapter VII, "True Stories about *Candida* and Related Diseases.")

People who eat a great deal of processed food may also be consuming many chemical preservatives or additives which can cause problems. Most canned and packaged dry and frozen foods, condiments and salad dressings, sauces and bouillon seasonings, contain chemicals. All hard cheeses contain chemicals, and soy cheese has far too many chemicals for the usually sensitive digestive system of the *Candida* patient.

All canned tomatoes and most other canned vegetables and potatoes contain citric acid as a preservative. In recipes it is preferable to use fresh tomatoes, vegetables, and potatoes instead of canned. Even common table salt contains chemicals; however sea salt has no chemicals and is recommended instead.

MSG (monosodium glutamate), a flavor enhancer, is in many foods, especially in most canned soups and other products. It has been known to cause headaches, chest pain, and other reactions. Be certain to check all labels to avoid this ingredient. Also, be aware that MSG is commonly used in Chinese food.

Molds

Many people have sensitivity to the molds that may be in their home or workplace. If the sensitivity becomes severe, steps must be taken to eliminate this irritant. If that is not possible, it may be necessary to find another home or workplace instead.

Clorox bleach has been successful in removing mold. However, gloves must be worn, and there should be enough ventilation during the mold-removal process. If a person is highly sensitive to mold, it would be better to have someone else remove the mold.

All hard cheeses are derived from mold and are therefore prohibited on the *Candida* Control Diet. In addition, mold can grow on coffee beans and tea leaves, as well as on dried herbs. Melons and skins of fruits and vegetables accumulate mold during their growth, so they should be cleaned well before peeling or cutting. Also, dried fruits collect mold during the drying process.

Mercury in Silver Amalgam Dental Fillings

Many cases of yeast syndrome are aggravated—if not actually caused—by the presence of mercury and other toxic metals in silver amalgam dental fillings. The label "silver amalgam" is misleading, because amalgams typically contain about 12% silver and 50% mercury, which is the most poisonous of the toxic metals.

Margery K., a woman in her late sixties, had been ill for many years since sewage seeped into her home during a flood. She began having bleeding sinuses and was diagnosed with *Candida* and CFS (Chronic Fatigue Syndrome).

I referred Margery to the book, *It's All in Your Head*, by Hal Huggins, DDS, who is an acknowledged leader in the field of alternative, holistic dentistry. She learned from Dr. Huggins' book how mercury and other toxic metals that are commonly used by dentists can cause sinusitis as well as fatigue, yeast overgrowth, and a whole host of other problems associated with heavy metal toxicity.

Ordinary blood and urine tests are usually not good indicators of mercury toxicity, so Margery had herself tested with something more specialized, called the Mercury Challenge Test. Her mercury level was very high, so she immediately made arrangements to travel from San Francisco to Colorado Springs to have Dr. Huggins remove and replace her amalgam fillings. Unfortunately, because Margery lived so far away, she had Dr. Huggins remove all of her amalgam fillings at one time. As a result, she had a very bad reaction. Her arms and legs broke out in the most terrible sores I had ever seen!

Margery also detoxified with supplements and Chelation Therapy. Over a period of several months, her health greatly improved. Her *Candida*, CFS, and sinus problems also cleared up.

CAUTION: See page 41. To prevent bad reactions, have these fillings replaced by a dentist who specializes in silver amalgam removal and will tailor the removal protocol to fit your needs. Connecticut dentist Mark Breiner, auhor of Whole Body Dentistry *is one.*

Parasites

It amazed me that so many of my support group members and those I counseled individually had parasites as well as *Candida* and related conditions. It is not known whether *Candida* causes the parasites to proliferate or if parasites cause the *Candida*. Nevertheless, parasites are a complicating factor in *Candida* recovery, and they must be addressed.

Many times a person has been diagnosed with parasites and received treatment, but never has been retested, which is a big mistake, because he/she may not have gotten completely rid of them. I have seen many cases in which patients have unknowingly been harboring parasites for years!

Parasites have been known to cause Irritable Bowel Syndrome (IBS), chronic fatigue, extreme diarrhea, constipation, allergies, depression, gastrointestinal cramps, bloating, gas, nausea, vomiting, weight loss, insomnia, lassitude, dizziness, muscle and joint pains, arthritic/rheumatoid symptoms, and much more.

A few years ago I received a letter from a woman in Africa. She and her family had been living there for two years because of her husband's job. She, her husband, and children had been ill since almost the day they arrived. They all experienced extreme fatigue, recurring throat infections, bouts of diarrhea and many other health problems.

Because the woman and her family were living in a foreign country and being subjected to foods and water to which they were unaccustomed, I suggested that they might have parasites, and that it would be beneficial for them to contact a doctor there, to be tested for them.

Just a couple of months later, the woman wrote again, to thank me, and tell me that a doctor diagnosed her whole family as having parasites and that, after receiving treatment for them, all of their symptoms disappeared.

You don't have to travel to other countries to get parasites today. You can easily acquire them right here in the U.S., by eating at any restaurant. This is usually because people who prepare salads or the salad bar may not have washed their hands thoroughly or cleaned the vegetables and fruit properly.

Organic fruits and vegetables, especially, have to be cleaned well. Not being treated with chemicals means that they can easily harbor parasites. So, the skins of any fruits and vegetables need to be scrubbed well before cutting.

Also, meat, poultry, and fish in restaurants can contain parasites if they are not cooked thoroughly. At home, it is wise to not only cook meat, poultry, and fish thoroughly, but to not cook them when they are fresh, as they can often harbor parasites. It is better to freeze them first before preparing them.

If a person has gone backpacking or swam in or ingested contaminated water, he or she could have obtained parasites. It is very easy to get Giardia parasites from water that has not been filtered or purified.

Ann Louise Gittleman's book, *Guess What Came to Dinner; Parasites and Your Health*, describes the problems of parasites in detail and is highly recommended.

Helicobacter (H. Pylori) is a bacterium that also comes from contaminated water. H. Pylori has been known to affect the intestines and cause gastritis, as well as to eventually lead to ulcers in the stomach and duodenum. It is important for people who have traveled outside of the U.S., especially, to be tested for H. Pylori. This can be done through blood and stool tests, as well as from biopsies.

Too Much Sugar/Complex Carbohydrates

When people have too much sugar in their diet it can cause the normally harmless *Candida albicans* yeast to become active and multiply. That causes symptoms from head to toe. *Candida albicans* thrive on all sugars, sweeteners, natural sugars in fruits and fruit juices, as well as too many complex carbohydrates.

If a woman has a yeast infection, after being tested by the doctor and receiving antiyeast/antifungal medication, the healthcare practitioner usually doesn't tell the patient that she should also treat herself internally by avoiding a high sugar/complex carbohydrate diet. It would be beneficial for her to be on the *Candida* Control Diet, which is described in more detail in *The Candida Control Cookbook*.

Men who have jock itch or athlete's foot should also avoid all sugars and too many complex carbohydrates, which can cause the yeast or fungal infection to continue or spread.

Stress

Dr. Bernie Siegel, cancer specialist and surgeon, wrote in his book, *Love, Medicine and Miracles,* "There is now experimental evidence that 'passive emotions,' such as grief, feelings of failure, and suppression of anger produce oversecretion of these same hormones, which suppress the immune system. The salient point is that our state of mind has an immediate and direct effect on any state of body."

This is further emphasized in the book, *Your Body Believes Every Word You Say: The Language of the Body /Mind Connection, 2nd ed.,* by Barbara Hoberman Levine.

III. Self-Help *Candida* Evaluations

Were You Exposed to *Candida*-Causing Factors?
1. Did you ever have a disease in the past? Presently?
2. Have you taken antibiotics?
3. If so, did you take them for a long time? Repeatedly?
4. Have you taken steroids, such as cortisone or prednisone?
5. If so, did you take them for a long time? Repeatedly?
6. Have you taken prescribed medications?
7. If so, did you take them for a long time? Repeatedly?
8. Have you taken antidepressant drugs?
9. If so, did you take them for a long time?
10. Have you taken estrogen or other hormones?
11. If so, did you take them for a long time?
12. Have you been subjected to mold or chemicals in your home or workplace?
13. Have you eaten a great deal of processed foods that contain chemicals, such as preservatives or additives?
14. Have you ever suffered physical injury?
15. Have you had any surgery?
16. Has your sexual partner been infected with *Candida*?
17. Have you received any implants?
18. Have you received radiation?
19. Have you had chemotherapy?
20. Have you suffered emotional trauma?
21. Have you had excessive or continual stress?

22. Have you eaten a diet that is high in sugar and sweeteners?
23. Have you eaten a diet that is high in complex carbohy-drates (breads and bakery items, cereals, pastas, pota-toes, rice)?
24. Have you ever had parasites?
25. Do you have silver amalgam fillings in your mouth?

NOTE: If you have been exposed to any of the above factors, you could have Candida, *a yeast infection.*

Have You Been Infected with a Disease or an Autoimmune Disorder?

ADD/ADHD
AIDS
ALS (Lou Gehrig's disease)
Acne
Alzheimer's disease
Asthma
Autism
Cancer
Cardiovascular disease
Celiac sprue
Chronic fatigue syndrome
Colitis
Crohn's disease
Cystitis
Diabetes
Eczema
Endometriosis
Epstein-Barr virus
Fibromyalgia
Gastritis
Gastroenteritis
Graves' disease
HIV
Hepatitis
Hodgkin's disease

Hypoglycemia
Mitral valve prolapse
Mononucleosis
Multiple sclerosis
Myasthenia gravis
Neurological disease
Osteoarthritis
Ovarian cysts
Parkinson's disease
Pelvic inflammatory disease
Psoriasis
Pulmonary disease
Rheumatic fever
Rheumatoid arthritis
Scleroderma
Shingles
Sinusitis
Thrush
Thyroid disease
Tuberculosis
Urethritis
Urticaria
Vaginitis
Vulvodenia

NOTE: If you have been infected with any of the above or another illness, you could have Candida. *(See why in Chapter II: "Candida-Causing Factors; Diseases and Autoimmune Disorders")*

Do You Have *Candida*-Related Symptoms?

Abdominal pains
Adrenal dysfunction
Allergies
Anxiety
Arethemia
Athlete's foot
Bad breath
Balance, loss of
Bloating after eating
Body odor
Breast soreness/pain
Breath, shortness of
Chemical sensitivity
Chest pains/tightness
Concentration problems
Constipation
Cough, persistent
Cravings for sweets
Depression
Diarrhea
Dizziness
Drowsiness, unusual
Dry feet
Ear infections
Energy loss
Eye burning/itching
Fatigue, extreme
Food sensitivity
Gas/bloating
Hair loss
Headaches
Heartburn
Hormone dysfunction
Hyperactivity
Hypoglycemia
Indigestion

Infertility
Insomnia
Irritability
Irritable bowel
Jaw pain, unexplained
Jock itch
Lack of energy
Leaky gut
Memory lapses
Migraines
Mold sensitivity
Mouth dryness/soreness
Mucus in stools
Muscle and joint pains
Nail fungus
Numbness/tingling
Odor sensitivity
PMS
Panic attacks
Rectal itch
Sexual dysfunction
Sinus infections
Skin rashes/itching
Spastic colon
Stomach bloating
Suicidal feelings
Tachycardia
Throat dryness/soreness
Thyroid dysfunction
Tinnitus
Urinary infections,
 frequency/urgency
Vaginal infections
Wheezing
White-coated tongue

If You Had Treatment but Didn't Recover

1. Did you follow the *Candida* Treatment Program precisely?
2. Did you follow the *Candida* Control Diet consistently and long enough?
3. Did you alternate the same foods, not less than 4 days apart?
4. Were you tested for food allergies?
5. Did you take antiyeast/antifungal medication?
6. If so, did you take it consistently and for long enough?
7. Did you take more than one antiyeast/antifungal medication at a time?
8. Did you take a natural antiyeast/antifungal product?
9. If so, did you take it consistently and for long enough?
10. Did you take more than one natural antiyeast/antifungal product at a time?
11. Did you take acidophilus, vitamin C, and other supplements to rebuild your immune system?
12. If so, did you take them consistently and long enough?
13. Have you been tested for thyroid dysfunction?
14. Have you been tested for adrenal gland dysfunction?
15. Did you ever travel outside of the U.S.?
16. Did you ever go backpacking, or swim in or drink water that was contaminated?
17. Have you eaten in restaurants often?
18. Have you prepared and cooked fresh meat, fish, and poultry?
19. Have you often eaten red meat and poultry that was not free of hormones or antibiotics?
20. Were you ever tested for parasites?
21. If so, and if you tested positive and had treatment, did you get rid of the parasites completely?

22. Were you ever retested for parasites?
23. Were you tested for allergy to mold, chemicals, and foods?
24. Were you tested for allergy to *Candida albicans*?
25. Were you tested for secretory IgA (enough saliva)?
26. Silver amalgams contain 50% mercury. Do you have any silver amalgam dental fillings? Many?
27. Were you ever tested for mercury poisoning?
28. If so, did you have any silver amalgams removed?
29. Is your diet high in sugars, sweeteners, and complex carbohydrates?
30. Have you taken any antibiotics or steroids since *Candida* treatment?
31. Have you taken any steroids, such as prednisone, cortisone, etc?
32. Have you taken pain medications? For a long time?
33. Have you taken anti-inflammatory drugs?
34. Have you taken diuretics?
35. Have you taken antidepressants?
36. Have you taken estrogen or other hormones?
37. Have you taken birth-control pills?
38. Have you taken many antacids?
39. Have you been under stress at work or home?
40. If so, has the stress been excessive or continued?
41. If you have reoccurring yeast infections, could your partner be reinfecting you?

IV. Why *Candida* Sufferers May Not Recover

Inconsistent Use of the *Candida* Control Diet

Many times *Candida* sufferers don't follow the *Candida* Control Diet precisely, consistently, and for a long enough period of time. Often when people feel better while they are on the diet, they tend to go off it too quickly.

Also, people have a difficult time staying on the diet; they relapse because it is so restrictive. Often they don't understand the need for its limitations, the importance of staying on the diet, or the many substitutions that are available for problem foods or ingredients.

It has been found that it is beneficial to stay on the diet until optimum health has been reached and then to still be careful by avoiding too many sugars or complex carbohydrates, or fruits, to prevent *Candida's* return.

The Candida Control Cookbook, which I also wrote, goes into great detail about the importance of the *Candida* Control Diet, and is written especially to appeal to the *Candida* sufferer, who usually feels very deprived. The cookbook contains more than 150 delicious recipes with tasty substitutions for problem ingredients and helps the individual to stay on the diet more easily.

Many *Candida* sufferers make the mistake of not alternating their foods on the diet, and they repeat the same food more often than four days apart. If they have a food or ingredient too often, they could easily develop an allergy to it, because the digestive system of the *Candida* victim is usually quite sensitive.

Incorrect Antiyeast/Antifungal Therapy

The *Candida* patient may not have taken the proper prescribed or natural antiyeast/antifungal for his or her particular type of condition, or perhaps the patient did not take it consistently and long enough, or perhaps more than one therapy was taken at a time.

It has been found that many *Candida* sufferers become so desperate to become well that they do more than one therapy and sometimes take many natural supplements during the same period of treatment, causing great complications in their recovery. It is therefore beneficial to take only one remedy at a time.

Inadequate Immune System Builders

When people have *Candida* or CRC, they usually have weakened immune systems. When the immune system is suppressed, it is prone to more infection and disease, making it impossible for a person to fully recover. (See Chapter V, "The *Candida* Treatment Program: Rebuild the Immune System.")

If a *Candida* sufferer doesn't realize the necessity for improving the immune system, he or she won't take adequate immune builders consistently and for a long enough time. ("See Appendix A—Supplements for *Candida* and the Immune System.")

Adrenal Gland Dysfunction

Adrenal gland dysfunction can create a complication to *Candida* recovery.

There are some health care professionals today who test for adrenal gland dysfunction. One such professional is Dr. Adiel

Tel-Oren[1], of Minneapolis, Minnesota. He is a chiropractic physician, a European medical doctor, a licensed Certified Clinical Nutritionist, as well as Diplomat of the American Chiropractic Board of Nutrition and the American Board of Oxidative Medicine.

Dr. Tel-Oren states, "Adrenal dysfunction can affect the immune system, which in turn can promote *Candida*." To test the adrenal system, Dr. Tel-Oren does the Adrenal Stress Index test, which measures the salivary levels of DHEA and cortisol throughout the day. These major hormones are actively involved in the body's development, growth, immune capabilities, and response to stress. They demonstrate the patient's "stress handling" capacity, in general, and specific biological functions in particular.

Lack of Hydrochloric Acid

If a person isn't digesting food properly, chances are that the antiyeast/antifungal, immune-building supplements, and other nutrients necessary for recovery are not being digested either. If this is the case, there could be a lack of hydrochloric acid, which is necessary for digestion. Stomach acids are important for activating various digestive enzymes and for protecting the body from pathological microorganisms that enter the mouth.

Many times *Candida*, as well as a person's aging, have been known to cause a lack of hydrochloric acid. Products designed to assist stomach digestion, which include hydrochloric acid, are

[1] To contact Dr. Tel-Oren, owner and director of Integrated HealthCare Clinics, Inc.
  Address: 2409 Lyndale Ave. South, Minneapolis, MN 55405
  Phone: (612) 870-2974
  Website: www.integratedhealthcare.org

available at holistic clinics, health and natural foods stores, and co-ops.

Lack of Pancreatic Enzymes

As mentioned above, insufficient digestion can lead to malabsorption, nutritional deficiencies, and the inability to benefit from nutritional therapies. Incomplete digestion can also result in fermentation of partially digested food particles, leading to increased toxicity of the gastrointestinal tract and the possibility of leaky gut syndrome. This can create an imbalance in the microflora of the gut, allowing *Candida* sufferers to persist in their dysfunctional state. Pancreatic enzymes are available in holistic clinics, health and natural foods stores, and co-ops.

Thyroid Dysfunction

Thyroid dysfunction, such as hypothyroidism (low thyroid) and hyperthyroidism (high thyroid), often goes hand-in-hand with *Candida*. It may be that *Candida* causes the thyroid gland to malfunction or vice versa.

When a person's temperature is usually low it may indicate hypothyroidism, so the person should contact a health care professional for testing. Many physicians test only TSH and T4 thyroid. But it has been found to be far more advantageous for a patient to have a full-panel thyroid test, which many traditional doctors are reluctant to order. They prefer, instead, to rely on the TSH and T4 testing, which does not always give a full picture of thyroid function.

Even though thyroid testing may show hypothyroidism or that the thyroid is in the normal range, the patient may still have Wilson's syndrome. E. Denis Wilson, M.D. describes this condition in his book, *Wilson's Syndrome: The Miracle of Feeling Well.*[2] This condition causes symptoms characteristic of hypothyroidism. It is characterized by a body temperature that runs, on average, below normal, while routine thyroid blood tests are often in the normal range. When temperatures are normalized with T3 therapy, the symptoms usually disappear. The temperature and symptoms generally remain improved even after treatment has been discontinued.

Many times, it has been found that once the thyroid is corrected, *Candida,* chronic fatigue syndrome, PMS, migraine headaches, spastic colon, irritable bowel syndrome, fibromyalgia, lupus, and many other conditions also improve.

Food, Environmental, and Chemical Sensitivities/Allergies

When food or chemical sensitivity exists, the protective and absorptive functions of the gastrointestinal tract become ineffective, as seen in infections (such as *Candidiasis*), in leaky gut syndrome, in overuse of certain drugs, (i.e., Tylenol, aspirin and ibuprofen), and in deficient immune state. The term "allergy" refers only to specific immunological reactions that are difficult to ascertain directly and accurately by current testing methods. These methods will not reveal nonallergic responses of the immune system.

On the other hand, the term "sensitivity" refers to all adverse reactions to the ingestion of foods or exposure to chemicals, including allergic, toxic, metabolic, genetic, and pharmacological

[2] To order the book, contact E. Denis Wilson, M.D., Wilson Syndrome Foundation, P.O. Box 539, Summerfield, FL 34492
Phone: 800-621-7006
Website: www.wilsonssyndrome.com

reactions. Therefore, testing for sensitivities is far more useful than testing merely for allergies.

The ALCAT test is a revolutionary test that accurately measures changes in the appearance and function of various blood components in response to foods, molds (including *Candida),* environmental chemicals, and food additives.

The ALCAT test[3] is also an effective tool for measuring effects of *Candida* on the immune system. This test has been investigated with double-blind experiments, and was found to have a high degree of correlation with clinical symptoms. People with conditions related to environmental and food sensitivities, such as migraine headaches, skin disorders, breathing problems, intestinal disorders, fatigue, hyperactivity, food cravings, and weight gain have demonstrated significant clinical improvement by limiting or eliminating the offending substances from their diet.

Dr. Tel-Oren has created new panels for the laboratory that provides the ALCAT test, to improve its cost-effectiveness for different types of patients. He can order the test directly through his office. He is also available to consult with other physicians and health care practitioners on how to order the test for the benefit of their patients.

Secretory IgA

This is an important immune component secreted by the gastrointestinal lining to fend off infections by yeast, bacteria, or parasites. According to Dr. Tel-Oren, the excretory IgA level can be revealed by a simple stool test.

---

[3] For more information see footnote 1 on page 21.

Colon Dysfunction

Some *Candida* sufferers try various antiyeast/antifungal agents to no avail. Their failure to heal may be caused by impacted fecal matter in the colon, which frequently occurs in our society. This problem results from improper diet, drug overuse, alcohol and caffeine consumption, chronic constipation, and other factors previously discussed in this chapter.

Impacted fecal material can harbor infectious microorganisms (fungus/yeast, bacteria, and parasites), leading to release of toxins and putrefactive products. Additionally, a thick and impermeable impaction may prevent antiyeast/antifungal remedies or drugs from reaching their targets, thus protecting the fungus and allowing the infection to persist. Some people unknowingly carry with them many unwanted pounds of impacted feces.

Colonic Hydrotherapy[4] is an effective approach to cleansing the entire large intestine of impacted fecal material, especially when it is "hidden" in commonly occurring "pockets" that protrude out of the colon (known as *diverticula*). When done appropriately, using state-of-the-art technology, following correct hygiene and sterilization, colonic hydrotherapy can complement other therapies to improve the hygiene and function of the entire colon and increase the likelihood of success when using antifungal, antibacterial, or antiparasitic agents.

Dr. Tel-Oren, who frequently recommends this therapy to his patients, states that his patients' success rate with infections and conditions of the colon have dramatically increased since a sophisticated colonic hydrotherapy system was installed in his offices and his patients have been treated with it.[5]

---

[4] See note 1 on page 21.
[5] See note 1.

Parasites

Many people have parasites along with *Candida*. Self-test parasite stool kits, available at many health care professionals' offices, have often been found to be inaccurate, because parasites usually live in the small intestines, rather than the stools.

A test that has been known to be more precise is the anoscopy or Rectal Swab Test. For this test, the physician uses a long cotton swab to collect fluid from the mucosa, high up in the rectum. However, it is usually difficult to find a physician who will perform this test.

Once parasites are confirmed, Flagyl, an antibiotic, is usually prescribed. However, it has been found that this medication can cause toxic effects in many patients, as well as *Candida* overgrowth. Natural parasite remedies, such as black walnut, citrus seed extract, and artemisia, have been found to be effective, and cause fewer reactions.

If a person thinks he or she may have parasites and takes a natural parasite remedy that gets rid of all the symptoms, then parasites obviously were the culprits.

V. The *Candida* Treatment Program

Antiyeast/Antifungal to Kill the Infection

There are prescription antiyeast/antifungals, such as Diflucan (also known as Fluconizole), Nystatin, Nizoral,[6] or Mycostatin to eliminate yeast or fungal infection. There are also many natural antiyeast/antifungals that do the job. These items are available in health and natural foods stores, and co-ops.

Garlic is also a known antiyeast/antifungal. Fresh garlic is very beneficial. However, during cooking or standard processing, the allicin—the principal substance in garlic—dissipates quickly. Many brands of odorless garlic pills are available in health and natural foods stores, and co-ops.

For more information on natural antiyeast/antifungals, see Appendix A—"Supplements for *Candida* and the Immune System."

Rebuild the Immune System

The following information is from the book, *The Garden Within: Acidophilus-Candida Connection,* by Keith Sehnert, M.D. "Acidophilus is known to be an excellent immune-system builder. However, acidophilus not only helps the immune system, but it inhibits and reduces *Candida* (yeast infection), produces hydrogen peroxide, as well as natural antibiotics, helps digest food and corrects digestive disorders."

Acidophilus capsules and powder, containing billions of good bacteria, have been known to be more potent and beneficial than the acidophilus in milk and yogurt.

Vitamin C is known to be another good immune builder. For

---

[6] Caution: Nizoral may be harmful to the liver.

those people who have sensitive digestive systems, Ester-C® has been found to be easier to digest than regular vitamin C, because it is naturally buffered, and it can also be absorbed more easily.

Pau D'Arco, an herb, also has been known to support the immune system. It is extracted from the inner bark of the tropical Pau D'Arco tree and is rich in lapachol, a chemical that promotes immune system health. Lapachol also aids the body in dealing with yeast/fungal infections. Pau D'Arco is produced as a tea, and it also comes in capsules as well as tinctures.

All of the above products are available in health and natural foods stores, and co-ops.

Other supplements that have been known to be helpful for the immune system are described in Appendix A—"Supplements for *Candida* and the Immune System."

The *Candida* Control Diet

This diet is necessary for recovery because certain foods promote yeast growth and may undo any good the antiyeast/antifungal might accomplish. Therefore, for the treatment program to be successful, this diet should be followed precisely and consistently.

Because the special diet may appear to be unduly strict, the reasons for its severity should be known to the sufferer, so that he or she is less likely to become discouraged and go off it. Although there are many problem and prohibited foods on the *Candida* Control Diet, there are also many permitted foods. *The Candida Control Cookbook,* which I also wrote, is based upon the *Candida* Control Diet.

When a person has *Candida*, he or she may not feel up to doing a lot of preparation and cooking. Therefore, *The Candida*

Control Cookbook has many delicious, easy-to-prepare meals. There are also numerous tips on easy snacks and even how to order safely when dining out.

Sugars, Sweeteners, and Complex Carbohydrates

One of the main purposes of the *Candida* Control Diet is to keep the sugars and complex carbohydrates low, to starve the yeast, especially in the beginning stages of treatment. Therefore, it is recommended that *Candida* sufferers keep their carbohydrate intake between 60 and 100 grams daily.

NOTE: It is recommended that a health care professional be consulted before you attempt the Candida *Control Diet.*

Not only sugar, but also most sweeteners should be avoided, because the *Candida albicans* yeast thrives on them. This includes dextrose, fructose, corn syrup, maltose, glucose, sorbitol, aspartame, saccharine, NutraSweet, Sweet'N Low, and any kind of malt, molasses, and honey. Soda pop contains high-fructose corn syrup and should be avoided. Be certain to read all labels, to avoid all sugars and sweeteners.

Fruits and Fruit Juices

All fruits contain too much natural sugar for the person who has *Candida*. Sadly, it has been found that some people, who seem to recover and then eat fruit, have symptoms return.

Fruit juice not only has natural sugar, but once fresh juice is opened and poured, yeast develops almost immediately. Be certain to read all labels to avoid "Sweetened with fruit juices." Rice cakes are permitted on the *Candida* Control Diet, but many of them are sweetened with fruit juices, or tamari, which should also be avoided.

In addition, dried fruits should be avoided, because of the mold that can grow during the drying process.

Dried Herbs, Coffees, and Teas

Dried herbs should be avoided, due to mold that can adhere to them in their drying process. It is better to use fresh herbs instead.

Coffees and teas should also be avoided because of the mold that can collect on coffee beans and tea leaves during drying. However, Taheebo tea (also known as Pau D'Arco), La Pacho, Ipe Roxo, Tabeula, Tacoma, and Bow Stick teas are recommended. These teas are made from the bark of trees grown in the rain forests of South America that are free of fungus and mold. They have been known to be effective antiyeast/antifungals.

Dairy Products

Most dairy products, except eggs[7] and clarified butter, are forbidden on the diet, because they contain lactose, a milk sugar, upon which the yeast can thrive. An easy method of clarifying butter, which gets rid of the lactose, is explained in *The Candida Control Cookbook*. There are also many delicious dairy substitutes in the cookbook.

Fermented Drinks and Foods

Beverages that have been fermented should be avoided. These include beer (fermented with brewer's yeast), liquor (made from fermented potatoes or corn), wine (made from fermented grapes), and others.

Foods made with vinegar (salad dressings, mayonnaise,

---

[7] Be certain you are not allergic to eggs.

mustard, meat sauces, marinades, and pickled items), malt products, tamari, soy sauce, teriyaki, etc., are not permitted on the *Candida* Control Diet, because anything fermented can upset the usually sensitive digestive system of the *Candida* patient.

The Candida Control Cookbook goes into great detail on "problem foods" and gives many suggestions for "Permitted Foods."

Gluten in Wheat

Candida albicans yeast also thrives on gluten. Therefore, breads and bakery products with wheat, which contains gluten, should be avoided, as well as grains, pastas, and cereals made with wheat, especially during the beginning stages of treatment. Be certain to read all labels on packaged products to avoid wheat and gluten. *The Candida Control Cookbook* suggests many permitted breads, grains, pastas, and cereals.

Breads without Wheat or Yeast

French Meadow Bakery makes breads permitted on the *Candida* Control Diet, and does not have any yeast in its facility, because yeast is airborne and contaminates other breads. French Meadow specializes in the following without wheat or yeast:

Brown Rice Bread (100% organic, wheat/yeast-free)
European Rye Bread (100% organic, wheat/yeast-free)
Kamut Bread (100% organic, wheat/yeast-free)
Millet Bread (100% organic, wheat/yeast-free)
Sourdough[8] French Bread (100% organic, yeast-free)

---

[8] Sourdough does contain wheat, but the acidophilus in its starter has been known to have beneficial properties that aid in digestion of the wheat. It also contains valuable nutrients.

Spelt Bread, Bagels, and Pizza Crusts (100% organic
wheat/yeast-free)
Whole Grain Rye (100% organic, wheat/yeast-free)

NEWS FLASH!! French Meadow has just come out with
all-organic WOMAN'S BREAD, containing natural soy
isoflavones, which give women natural support throughout
PMS, menopause, and the postmenopausal years. Recommended
by many leading dieticians and health practitioners, this bread is
also beneficial for men. Another new item, organic HEALTH-
SEED SPELT BREAD (100% wheat-free), is high in protein,
flaxseed, and pumpkinseed.

*NOTE: French Meadow distributes the above items nation-
ally to health and natural foods stores, and co-ops. To order:
(877) NOYEAST or www.frenchmeadow.com Address: French
Meadow, 2610 Lyndale Ave. South, Minneapolis, MN 55408.*

Pacific Bakery™, "Home of the Yeast Free Guarantee," also
makes yeast-free breads. This bakery emphasizes that they are
the only yeast-free bread manufacturer that freshly stone-grinds
their own whole organic grains daily and makes all of their
bread in one facility in the USA. This bakery has a yeast-free
guarantee, because it never has yeast in its building, and the
owner maintains that it never will.

Also, all of Pacific Bakery's whole grain breads are just
that—not a blend with white flour. Of the many breads that Pacific makes, the two best-selling ones are: wheat alternative
whole grain Spelt and Kamut breads. Also, Pacific has "white"
Spelt and Kamut breads. These breads are organic; sugar, honey,
dairy, and egg free. They are also free of baking powder and
baking soda, and they are either fat free or low fat.

*NOTE: Pacific Bakery distributes and ships nationwide, in-
cluding Hawaii and Alaska. Ask for Pacific Bakery's yeast-free*

products at your local natural foods store. If they are not available, contact Pacific Bakery,

    Address: P.O. Box 950, Oceanside, California 92049

    Phone: 760-757-6020

    Website: www.pacificbakery.com

    CELIAC DISEASE PATIENTS PLEASE NOTE: All Pacific Bakery products contain naturally occurring gluten.

VI. How to Prevent *Candida*

Ensure a Healthy Immune System

It is extremely important to keep the immune system in good condition. Acidophilus, vitamin C, and other supplements have been found to be beneficial in accomplishing this. See Appendix A—"Supplements for *Candida* and the Immune System."

Medications

When medications such as antibiotics, steroids, anti-inflammatory and antidepressant drugs, diuretics, hormones and birth-control pills are prescribed for you, it may be beneficial to also take prescribed antiyeast/antifungals to avoid developing a yeast infection. These include Diflucan (Fluconizole), Nystatin, Mycostatin, and Nizoral *(Caution: Nizoral can cause liver damage).* The antiyeast/antifungal should not be taken at exactly the same time as the antibiotic or other medication; rather, at least one or two hours before or afterward.

If a doctor is not willing to prescribe an antiyeast/antifungal medication, then natural ones, such as odorless garlic pills, caprylic acid, etc. (from health and natural foods stores, and co-ops) could be taken.

When taking medications, it has also been found to be beneficial to take natural immune builders. (See Appendix A—"Supplements for *Candida* and the Immune System".) Immune builders should not be taken at exactly the same time as the medication; rather one or two hours before or afterward, and for at least two months after the drugs are finished.

Hormones

Estrogen has been known to depress the immune system and may cause endometrial cancer, heart disease, *Candida,* and other serious side effects. Progesterone, rather than estrogen, is necessary to build bones. It may be beneficial to use natural hormone replacements that should have fewer side effects.[9]

Antacids

Candida albicans yeast also thrives in an acid-free environment. All prescription and nonprescription antacids promote this type of environment, so they should be avoided. Charcoal capsules/tablets and bifidus can be used for stomach distress, instead. Hydrochloric acid (digestive enzymes) aids in digestion, and its acidification may reduce yeast levels.

Invasive Procedures

If you need to have surgery, implants, radiation, chemotherapy, etc., it is important to first build up your immune system with vitamin C, acidophilus, and other beneficial supplements. Then, when the invasive procedure occurs, your immune system will be prepared to withstand it. Immune-building supplements are listed in Appendix A—"Supplements for *Candida* and the Immune System."

Chemicals

Find out if there are harmful chemical in the cleaning and laundry products in your home. If they are there, get rid of them immediately! They can aggravate your problems if you are sensitive. Use

[9] The use of hormone replacement therapy is still being evaluated. Consult your doctor.

natural products instead; these are available at many natural foods stores and co-ops, and from companies that specialize in producing products that are free of harmful chemicals.

Some products in your home may not only irritate you, but could cause cancer if they contain propylene glycol, which is a potential carcinogen (cancer-causing) ingredient. Propylene glycol is an automatic brake and hydraulic fluid, industrial antifreeze, and a de-icer for airplanes.

Many leading cosmetic companies have used propylene glycol in their cosmetics and personal care products for years, because it glides easily over the skin and is inexpensive to produce. It also works as a humectant; that is, it retains and prevents the escape of moisture in skin and cosmetic products. Mineral oil contains propylene glycol.

The problem of propylene glycol being in cosmetics and personal hair and skin care products is that its molecules are so small that they can easily enter the skin and affect the brain or body organs. A safety data sheet put out by the U.S. government warns us to "Avoid skin contact with propylene glycol, as this strong skin irritant may cause liver dysfunction and kidney damage." The FDA has not done anything about this problem. Products containing propylene glycol are legally in use today because they were "grandfathered" into legality by the federal government many years ago.

The following personal hair-care products in your home may contain propylene glycol: shampoos, conditioners, foaming mousse stylers, hair-setting sprays, and finishing hair sprays. There are even harmful ingredients in some baby shampoos.

Propylene glycol can also be found in bubble baths, hand and body soaps, cosmetics, lotions, moisturizers, and shaving creams and gels. Even baby bubble baths can contain harmful ingredients. Be certain to read all labels to avoid this harmful chemical.

Dr. Samuel Epstein, a professor of Occupational and Environmental Medicine at the School of Public Health, University of Illinois Medical Center, is an internationally recognized authority on toxic and carcinogenic effects of the environment, and has been director of the Cancer Prevention Coalition. The author of 280 scientific articles and seven books, including *The Safe Shopper's Bible,* he has recommended cosmetics, hair care, and personal care products that are carcinogen-free.

It is important to read *A Cure for All Cancers*, by Hulda Regehr Clark, Ph.D., N.D. She wrote, "100% of cancer patients have the solvent propyl alcohol in their liver and in their cancerous tissue. Don't use anything that has 'prop' in the list of ingredients."

Another carcinogen is sodium lauryl sulfate (SLS), which is used in strong detergents and garage floor cleaners, as well as engine degreasers and auto cleaning products. It is known as a common skin irritant and can rapidly be absorbed by the eyes, brain, heart, and liver, which may result in harmful long-term effects.

SLS could retard healing, may cause cataracts in adults, and also may keep children's eyes from developing properly. SLS is used in many personal care products, and also is in most toothpaste that is sold in retail stores. It is even present in some "natural toothpaste," which is sold in health and natural foods stores, and co-ops.

Alcohol, which is also harmful, is a principal ingredient in most mouthwash products. It would be beneficial to purchase mouthwash that is made without alcohol.

Sodium laureth sulfate (SLES) is the alcohol form of SLS. It is slightly less irritating than SLS, but may cause more drying.

Both SLS and SLES may cause potentially carcinogenic formations of nitrates and dioxins to form in shampoos and cleansers by reacting with other product ingredients. Large amounts of nitrates may enter the blood system from just one shampooing with the above.

Be certain to read all labels to avoid these chemicals. If you are a beautician or manicurist, it would be very beneficial to change the products you use to those that are free of carcinogens and other harmful ingredients.

Aluminum has been suspected of causing Alzheimer's disease and breast cancer. It is found in most deodorants and antiperspirants that are on the market today. It is even in "natural deodorants" in health and natural foods stores. Be certain to read all labels to avoid aluminum.

To avoid chemicals in foods, it is best to avoid soy cheese, canned soups and vegetables—especially tomatoes and other processed foods, which usually contain citric acid and other preservatives. It is better to make homemade soups instead and use fresh or frozen vegetables.

Because MSG is used as a flavor enhancer in soups, condiments, and other processed foods, read labels carefully. Also, because it is commonly used in Chinese foods, when you go to a Chinese restaurant, tell the waiter that you don't want MSG used in your food. Most Chinese restaurants are very accommodating about this request.

Molds

To avoid harmful molds in your home, check especially in your basement, inside and around your air-conditioner, and beneath and behind your refrigerator.

Clorox bleach has been found to be beneficial in removing

molds. In using this product or any other mold remover, rubber gloves should be worn; if you are too sensitive to undertake this job, have someone else remove the mold when you are not present.

It also would be best to avoid hard cheeses, which are derived from mold.

Nursing Mothers and Babies

A nursing mother who has *Candida* can give the condition to her baby through her breast milk. To prevent infecting the baby, the doctor may prescribe Diflucan or Nystatin for the mother, and liquid Nystatin may be prescribed for the baby—both to prevent infection and to avoid reinfecting the mother.

Sexual Relations

Often, when a woman gets repeated vaginal yeast infections, it is because her partner is re-infecting her. Especially, if the immune system is weak, *Candida* may easily be obtained from an infected partner through sexual intercourse. It is advised that during the time of the infection, a condom be used. Kissing on the mouth and oral sex should be completely avoided as well.

Avoid a High Sugar/High Complex Carbohydrate Diet

Too much sugar and too many complex carbohydrates, such as pastas, rice, potatoes, cereals, breads and bakery products, and so on, can encourage the *Candida albicans* yeast to become active and harmful.

Even fruit and fruit juices should be consumed in moderation because they contain a great deal of natural sugar and can encourage *Candida*. Natural vitamin supplements may be taken instead. It is better to incorporate into your diet food that is healthful, such as a large amount of vegetables, grains, natural meats, poultry, fish, and nuts.[10]

Meats and Poultry

Meat and poultry which are grown with antibiotics and steroids should be avoided. Natural, organically grown meats and poultry are recommended instead. However, they do cost much more than those that are conventionally grown.

If natural meats and poultry are not affordable, there are healthful alternatives: fish, vegetables, grains without wheat-containing gluten, tofu,[11] and nuts. Many vegetarian recipes, with good substitutions for problem ingredients, are described in *The Candida Control Cookbook.*

Silver Amalgam Dental Fillings

Patients who need dental fillings can request that their dentist not use silver amalgam, because it contains 50% mercury and only about 12% silver. Mercury is the most poisonous of the toxic metals.

Patients may instead request that the dentist make the fillings out of a composite material. However, the patient should also insist on first being tested with the new material, to see if there is any sensitivity to it before having it as a replacement.

In addition, when a dentist removes a silver amalgam filling,

---

[10] If you have a sensitive digestive system, it may be beneficial to grind the nuts. Also, there are delicious, easy recipes for nut butters in *The Candida Control Cookbook.*

[11] Tofu is derived from soy. Make certain you are not sensitive to it.

a dental dam should be used in the mouth to prevent the patient from ingesting any mercury that escapes.

If the dentist is unwilling to use anything other than a silver amalgam filling, or to test for sensitivity to a different material, or to use caution in removing the filling, then it would be beneficial to find another dentist who will accommodate those safety measures.

The protocol to be followed for the removal of mercury fillings differs from patient to patient. The protocol is determined by their individual needs after a thorough health assessment.

The Removal of Silver Amalgams

by Leo B. Cashman, Minneapolis Health Writer

An impressive majority of people who have had toxic dental work replaced and then detoxified have benefited. A Seattle researcher, Dietrich Klinghardt, M.D., Ph.D., explains why. Klinghardt states that "Most, if not all, chronic infectious diseases (including fungal and viral illnesses) are not caused by a failure of the immune system, but occur as a conscious adaptation of the immune system to an otherwise lethal heavy metal environment."

To prevent nerve and other cells from being suffocated by mercury, the immune system cultivates a large population of fungi and bacteria, which are able to bind the toxic metals in their cell walls, enabling the patient's own cells to breathe. The downside of all this is that the patient's body must then deal with the undesirable side effects of the yeast and bacteria, with their toxic wastes.

In addition to having his own medical practice, Dr. Klinghardt teaches a detoxification protocol, known as "Neural Therapy" to other health practitioners. Others prominent in the field of heavy metal detoxification are Thomas Levy, M.D. and H.I. "Sam" Queen of Queen & Co., both of Colorado Springs. Dr. Levy has teamed up with holistic dentist Hal Huggins to write a new book entitled, *Uninformed Consent: The Hidden Dangers in Dental Care* (Hampton Roads, 1999), reporting on the serious role that "dental revision" and the detoxification process need to play in addressing health problems ranging from chronic fatigue, MS, ALS (Lou Gehrig's disease), lupus, and other immune disorders, to breast cancer, leukemia, depression, and Alzheimer's Disease.

It is best for the patient to become armed with information from books such as these before deciding on dental work options. It is advisable to seek care from a respected, experienced, holistic dentist so that the work can be done safely, according to the best protocol, and so that additional mercury exposure from the amalgam removal process can be minimized. DAMS Inc., a nonprofit educational organization, has further information on this subject.

NOTE: For information on locations of mercury-free dentists, call the national office of DAMS, Inc. (Dental Amalgam Mercury Syndrome) at 1-800-311-6265, or write to P.O. Box 7249, Minneapolis, Minnesota 55407. DAMS has many resources. Ask for an information packet and a list of practitioners in your area who are familiar with the dental-health issues discussed here.

Parasites

If you eat out in restaurants, avoid salads and salad bars. Fresh vegetables and fruits might not have been cleaned thoroughly, or food handlers many not have washed their hands properly. Order only well cooked meat, poultry, and fish. Also, avoid raw sushi.

At home do not cook, broil, or bake any fresh meat, poultry or fish. Instead, freeze meat and poultry for at least 24 hours, and freeze fish for at least 48 hours before preparation, to kill any parasites. In addition, after coming into contact with raw meat, poultry, or fish, wash your hands thoroughly with warm, soapy water, and scrub sharp knives or utensils, as well as cutting boards with Clorox bleach and hot water to prevent contamination.

When purchasing meats and poultry, place them in separate plastic bags from the grocery store, to prevent their juices from contaminating fruits and vegetables in your grocery cart or refrigerator at home.

Clean the skins of all fruits and vegetables thoroughly before peeling or slicing. Fruits and vegetables, especially organic ones, can be predisposed to parasites because they have no chemicals to protect them. These may also be soaked in food-grade peroxide or citrus seed extract to prevent parasites.

To avoid Giardia parasites, which can be in water, drink only filtered or purified water. If backpacking, take enough bottled water along, so no water is ingested from possibly contaminated places.

When traveling to other countries, it's wise to take along an antiparasite remedy as a prevention. Drink only bottled water and beverages, use only purified ice, do not brush your teeth with tap water, use bottled water instead. Also, avoid fresh fruits and vegetables, unless the skins are scrubbed well before peeling or slicing.

Stress

It may be time to take inventory of your relationships with your mate, children, parents, siblings, friends, and coworkers. If you are having stress in these relationships, it is beneficial to reduce the stress, as much as possible.

If you are working at a job that is causing you great stress, it is important that you reduce or remove this pressure. If that is impossible, try to obtain a different job, even if it means less pay. When your health is at stake, it is important to safeguard it at all costs.

If you cannot alleviate or remove the stress on your own, it is recommended that you seek professional counseling to help. If funds are a problem, there are counseling services available at reasonable rates through your county, Jewish Family Service, Catholic Services, and other religious agencies.

In addition, it is recommended that you contact Emotions Anonymous (EA),[12] a worldwide organization that has existed for many years. Their meetings are fashioned after Alcoholics Anonymous (AA) and its 12-Step Program.

A Positive Attitude

A positive attitude is one of the most valuable tools in recovering from or preventing *Candida* and related conditions.

Dr. Bernie Siegel, a cancer specialist and surgeon, found that a positive attitude helped his cancer patients to heal. In *Love, Medicine & Miracles*, Dr. Siegel showed that there was direct

---

[12] To find out about an EA support group in your area, call the EA International telephone number: 651-647-9712, or write to P.O. Box 4245, St. Paul, Minnesota 55104.

evidence of a connection between the immune system and the brain.

He wrote, "One of the most widely accepted explanations of cancer, the 'surveillance theory,' states that cancer cells are developing in our bodies all the time, but are normally destroyed by white blood cells before they develop into cancerous tumors.

"Cancer appears when the immune system becomes suppressed and can no longer deal with the routine threat. It follows that whatever upsets the brain's control of the immune system will foster malignancy. We can change the body by dealing with how we feel."

I highly recommend Dr. Siegel's books. Barbara Hoberman Levine further illustrates the importance of a positive attitude in healing oneself in her highly recommended book *Your Body Believes Every Word You Say: The Language of the Body/Mind Connection, 2nd ed.*

VII. True Stories about *Candida* and Related Diseases

Antibiotics Caused Allen's *Candida*

Allen W. had rheumatic fever when he was 8 years old. For 8 more years his doctor had him take antibiotics daily as a preventative against developing mitral valve prolapse. From childhood all the way into his early 50s, whenever he went to his dentist for cleanings and filling of cavities and other dental work, he was ordered by the dentist to take many doses of antibiotics to prevent possible heart-valve infection. The American Heart Association has made it mandatory for dentists to have patients with any heart damage to follow this antibiotic protocol prior to any dental work.

Because of the antibiotics, Allen had poor digestion, gas, bloating, belching, severe stomach cramping, nausea, vomiting, diarrhea, anxiety, and panic attacks. It was difficult for him to travel or go out socially, because he was afraid of getting sick, which resulted in his eventually becoming an agoraphobic.

After he developed gastrointestinal failure, I recommended that Allen see Dr. Keith Sehnert, an M.D. who also practices alternative care. He checked Allen's mouth and saw that he had thrush (a white-coated tongue), which is yeast infection, as well as dry feet, also typical of *Candida.* He not only diagnosed Allen with *Candida,* but also suspected he had hypothyroidism (low thyroid).

After confirming his diagnosis of *Candida,* Dr. Sehnert put Allen on the *Candida* Control Diet, which Allen followed by using *The Candida Control Cookbook.* He prescribed Diflucan, an antiyeast/antifungal medication, and recommended vitamin C, garlic, and acidophilus to help rebuild Allen's immune system. Hypothyroidism was also confirmed, so Dr. Sehnert prescribed Synthroid for him.

In addition, Allen took digestive enzymes to replace the hydrochloric acid he seemed to lack, and which is necessary to digest food properly. Dr. Sehnert also had him tested for food allergies; afterward, Allen began to avoid the foods toward which he showed sensitivity.

After only a few days of following this course of treatment, he noticed that his stomach cramping had lessened. Several weeks later, he experienced great improvement in his digestive and other symptoms.

Later, I encouraged Allen to see his internist for an echocardiogram test, to see if he did have a heart problem. Those test results showed that he didn't have any heart issue. His doctor said that Allen didn't need to take antibiotics anymore when he went for dental work, and gave him a note to that effect for his dentist.

Today, Allen seems to be enjoying good health. His anxiety and agoraphobia have decreased. He is still careful with his diet, trying to not eat any food that he knows could give him problems. However, when he occasionally eats sugar products, he does notice stomach gas. Other than that, he experiences none of the physical symptoms he did previously.

He recently told me that, when he has to take antibiotics for any infection, his *Candida* does return. However, he then takes Diflucan and acidophilus, not at exactly the same time as the antibiotic, but at least two hours afterward, which improves his *Candida* symptoms within two days. He seems to be doing very well with this regimen.

Many people get *Candida* due to the antibiotics that are routinely given to them. **It is time for them to ask their doctors if the antibiotics are really necessary.** If so, they need to also take an antiyeast/antifungal and immune builders to prevent yeast infection—not at exactly the same time, but at least two hours before or after the antibiotic.

Bob Had Great Determination to Recover

Bob P. is a member of my support group. I have also done individual counseling with him. He had had problems for years, ever since he lost his mother at age 6 and became an orphan when his father died soon after. His stepmother raised him, but was negligent and abusive.

When his paternal grandmother took him in for a while, she gave him all kinds of sugary bakery goods. As a result, he became obese, concentrated poorly in school, and became fatigued easily.

When he was 12, he experienced more problems with concentration, extreme fatigue and weakness, and attacks of depression and anxiety. Later, these conditions became worse, and he developed asthma.

Bob said, "As a college student, I had to push myself to accomplish anything. I wasn't feeling well mentally. I became very frustrated with my life, and went from being an intellectual to an underachiever. I desperately wanted to become successful, but did not know what was keeping me from accomplishing it. I knew something was wrong medically with me, but I couldn't figure it out. I felt lost!

"I became an alcoholic, was becoming all the more fatigued, and began sleeping for over 12 hours a day on a regular basis. I had great difficulty staying awake and greater difficulty holding a job. I was very depressed and had a good amount of anxiety, as well."

Bob sought medical help and was told that he had a chemical imbalance. He was given antidepressants, which made him sleep more than ever, and he also became extremely depressed. He realized that he needed to get a proper diagnosis of his condition, to begin achieving wellness.

Because his mother had diabetes, Bob had his blood sugar checked. However, the test showed that he had hypoglycemia (low blood sugar) instead. He read a book on hypoglycemia, by the Broda Barnes Foundation, which referred him to a well-known holistic physician. The doctor diagnosed Bob's condition as *Candida* and low thyroid, along with the hypoglycemia. (Often, hypoglycemia and thyroid dysfunction go hand-in-hand with *Candida*.) The doctor prescribed Nystatin, an antiyeast/antifungal, for the *Candida,* as well as medication for his thyroid. For the hypoglycemia, Bob was advised to avoid sugar and to eat more protein every three to four hours, instead.

Bob was also directed to the Carl Pfeiffer Treatment Center in Naperville, Illinois, where he was diagnosed with a histamine imbalance, and also inadequate levels of vitamin B6 and zinc. His doctor recommended nutrients for the histamine imbalance and the B6 and zinc he was lacking. He also began adhering to a strict diet of no alcohol, chocolate, caffeine, dairy, yeast, wheat, or sugars. His health improved dramatically. He eventually became a vegetarian, which enabled him to lose weight, and his health improved even more.

Later, Bob was able to attend a university, and his concentration level had improved so much that he maintained a B average. His energy level also increased, and he began to exercise regularly. He was able to have a modeling/acting career while also working for a worldwide religious organization.

When I last spoke with Bob a little over a year ago, he told me that he was enjoying a fairly healthful life. This was all due to his great determination to conquer *Candida,* as well as other related health problems, and achieve wellness.

Sarah Had Fibromyalgia Syndrome (FMS) and *Candida*

Sarah B., 48 years old, consumed many antibiotics over the years, to treat recurring bronchitis and other infections. As a result, she had extreme fatigue, poor digestion, bloating after eating, and "brain fog." She also had muscle and joint pains. Three months before we met, she had been diagnosed with FMS and was receiving steroids (cortisone shots) from her physician.

After attending my support group and learning that steroids could cause *Candida* as well as suppress the immune system, she wanted to find a natural health care professional who would use other methods of treatment.

When I referred her to such a professional, Sarah was diagnosed with *Candida* as well as fibromyalgia. Many *Candida* patients have fibromyalgia. She was placed on the *Candida* Treatment Program, which consisted of the *Candida* Control Diet, Diflucan, an antiyeast/antifungal, as well as acidophilus and vitamin C—immune builders.

Sarah purchased my book, *The Candida Control Cookbook*, to help her stay on the *Candida* Control Diet. It took about six months for her *Candida* to clear up. Her fibromyalgia symptoms improved as well.

Today, Sarah maintains that she is free of *Candida* and most of her fibromyalgia symptoms. However, she is still careful with her diet, staying away from sugar and wheat with gluten. However, she told me that if she ever has to take antibiotics or steroids, she will not do so unless she also takes an antifungal, as well as acidophilus and other immune builders during the same period.

I cautioned her to not take them at exactly the same time as the antibiotics, but at least two hours before or afterward.

Holly Suffered from *Candida* and Multiple Chemical Sensitivity (MCS)

Holly L., age 51, a *Candida* support group member and person I counseled, had been sick for several years and was diagnosed in 1994 with *Candida*. It is interesting to note that Holly's mother and some other close members of her family also had *Candida*.

When last we spoke Holly had not fully recovered from her *Candida* using the *Candida* Treatment Program because she didn't fully address her chemical sensitivities, or her other health problems. She had been exposed to many chemicals over several years while selling hair care products, cosmetics, and photocopy machines that used cartridges of harmful chemicals. Her home also had become a toxic environment from the mold that formed following the flooding of her basement. She was dealing with these issues when we last spoke.

Holly wanted my readers to know, "If a person doesn't adhere to the *Candida* Control Diet and eliminate food allergens for a long enough time to not tax the immune system and intestinal tract, and if the immune system isn't rebuilt, there will never be recovery."

Rosa's Family Wasn't Supportive

Rosa M., one of the people I counseled, was 26 years old and living at home with her parents. Rosa and her whole family were from Mexico. She suffered for many years with recurring vaginal infections, poor digestion, and extreme fatigue.

After she was diagnosed with *Candida* by her gynecologist, she started the *Candida* Control Diet. However, it was very difficult for her to stay on it, because her family didn't understand Rosa's condition. They constantly urged her to "eat their foods," much to her detriment.

Rosa needed to be around people who were more supportive. I encouraged her to attend a *Candida* support group, where she could be with other people who had similar health problems.

I also encouraged her to follow the *Candida* Control Diet by purchasing *The Candida Control Cookbook.* I also referred her to a physician who understood *Candida* and would prescribe Diflucan. Diflucan is an antiyeast/antifungal that has been effective in the treatment of *Candida,* with very few side effects.

Rosa had also developed a rash on her hands, which her doctor diagnosed as a fungal infection. He had thought that Diflucan would take care of it. However, it was not helping the rash.

I told Rosa that Taheebo Tea, a natural antiyeast/antifungal, had been found to be beneficial in getting rid of *Candida.* It has also been known to help relieve body rashes, when used as a compress. To make the compress, after the tea is brewed and cooled, a cloth is soaked in it and patted over the rash. I suggested that if Rosa also soaked her hands in the cooled tea, she might get some relief. She did this, and her rash cleared up very quickly.

I also suggested to Rosa that she talk with her family about her condition. She needed to tell them that she has a medical condition that could become very serious, and that if she eats their food, she will get terribly sick.

It is typical for people who have *Candida* to not get any support from family and friends. Their lack of understanding is usually because of their unfamiliarity with *Candida.* In addition, to some people a yeast infection in others may seem minor. It may also seem unlikely to them that a *Candida* sufferer can have so many different common symptoms and yet have to be on a special diet to get rid of them.

If this is happening to you, it is very important that you first try to teach the people close to you that *Candida* can become a serious medical condition. If they still do not understand, surround yourself with positive people instead—ones who will be very supportive of your condition and the special diet you need to recover.

If you don't have any positive, supportive family or friends, you can get a great deal of support from members of a *Candida* support group. If you don't have such a group in your area, see Chapter IX—"How to Start a Candida Support Group."

Rachael Suffered with Lupus and *Candida*

Rachael B., a 43-year-old woman I also counseled, had been ill for many years with systemic lupus. She said that she had experienced extreme fatigue, muscle and joint pains, skin rash, bloating, and diarrhea. She also had nephritis. In addition, she suffered greatly from reoccurring yeast infections, which she learned were caused by many rounds of antibiotics, as well as the prednisone she routinely took for the lupus.

She told me that she was going to see a natural health care professional, who was also an M.D., and that he had been extremely successful in treating *Candida.*

Subsequent to her office visit, she relayed that the doctor diagnosed her with chronic *Candidiasis,* as well as lupus, and he put her on the *Candida* Control Diet and Nystatin.

When she had been on Nystatin treatment for two months, and after she had been on the special diet for approximately six months, she informed me that not only did the yeast infections clear up, but also, her lupus symptoms improved significantly.

It is not unusual for people who suffer major disease to show improvement, as well as to control their *Candida* after being on an antiyeast/antifungal and following the *Candida* Control Diet. As a matter of fact, improvement from this form of treatment has been seen many times, not only in lupus patients, but also in those who have AIDS, cancer, multiple sclerosis, rheumatoid arthritis, and many other autoimmune diseases.

Brenda's Chronic Fatigue Syndrome (CFS) and *Candida*

Brenda J. was a "Wonder Mom." She held a job as executive secretary for a major insurance firm and worked for two executives there. However, they had moved in three more from the field, and she now found herself working for five executives who demanded a great deal of her time. She never took breaks and often worked overtime. In addition, she managed a large home and two families, because she had remarried two years previously.

She began to have repeated urinary tract infections, which were treated with rounds of antibiotics. Then she developed a stomach condition, with cramps and diarrhea. She was diagnosed with irritable bowel syndrome (IBS) and given many medications: Librax, Librium, and Immodium. She also became extremely tired and depressed.

She came to see me for counseling and told me, "There were times when I would come home after work at night and cry at the drop of a hat! Also, I was so exhausted that when I would be drying dishes, it seemed that my hands were not connected to me." Other doctors had diagnosed her with Chronic Fatigue Syndrome (CFS).

She confided to me that her stomach was so bloated that she was embarrassed to go out socially. In addition, her memory was poor, and many times her husband would have to finish a sentence for her, or come up with a common word that she had forgotten. Stomach bloating and poor memory are typical *Candida* symptoms, and I suspected that she had that condition, as well as CFS.

I informed her that *Candida* can be related to CFS and recommended she see a health care professional familiar with it. She followed my advice, and the doctor confirmed that she had *Candida*. He prescribed Diflucan, the *Candida* Control Diet, acidophilus, and other supplements to rebuild her immune system.

About eight months later, her *Candida* was controlled and her CFS showed dramatic improvement, as well.

Claire's Multiple Sclerosis (MS) Improved with *Candida* Therapy

Claire F., another person I counseled, had been diagnosed with MS several years before. She suffered with numbness, tingling, and muscle weakness, as well as poor memory. She also had poor digestion and reoccurring vaginal yeast infections.

Eventually she had to use a cane—and an electric cart whenever she did shopping in grocery or department stores.

I recommended a health care practitioner, who diagnosed her as having *Candida* as well as MS. He prescribed Diflucan, an antiyeast/antifungal, and instructed her to go on the *Candida* Control Diet.

The Diflucan and special diet helped her *Candida* symptoms improve. However, it was difficult for her to stay on the diet, because it was so restrictive, and her symptoms returned. I suggested that she try *The Candida Control Cookbook*, which she did, and it made it much easier for her to stay on the diet.

Once she followed the diet faithfully, her yeast infections, as well as her MS symptoms began to improve. This has been found to happen among many other MS patients.

Claire stayed on the diet persistently for over a year. However, when she went off it and ate a great deal of carbohydrates, her symptoms returned. She told me that she had terrible cravings for sugary foods. This is typical of *Candida* sufferers, because many times it's the yeast that's craving the sweets. I told her that Chromium Picolinate™ had been found to be helpful in controlling sugar cravings, as well as hypoglycemia (low blood sugar). She purchased that product and thought it helped her cravings a great deal.

She stayed on the *Candida* Control Diet for three more years, until about a year ago. To this day, her *Candida* is controlled and her MS is significantly improved.

Roger Had AIDS, and Suffered Greatly with *Candida*

Roger K. was a member of my support group because he wanted to find out more about *Candida*. He had been diagnosed with AIDS a few years before. However, he had also suffered greatly with thrush which is a yeast infection, in his throat and esophagus. Thrush is a typical problem of many AIDS patients.

Robert was treated for *Candida* with Nystatin, an antiyeast/antifungal, and went on the *Candida* Control Diet. He told me that, after a few weeks, his throat and esophagus began to heal, and he felt much better. Also, after a few months, his T-Cells greatly improved. This is not uncommon; AIDS patients and patients with different autoimmune diseases have also shown improvement with antiyeast/antifungal treatment.

When there is major disease or autoimmune disorders, infections can easily occur. Then antibiotics are prescribed, as they were for Roger. The antibiotics can easily cause *Candida*. Often patients suffer more from *Candida* symptoms than from their "primary" disease.

When a person has a disease or autoimmune disorder, their immune system becomes compromised. When this happens, the usually harmless *Candida albicans* yeast becomes active. The yeast can produce toxins, which have been known to invade the brain, mouth, esophagus, and intestines, and travel all the way to the colon, wreaking havoc along the way. (This information can't be stressed enough.)

It is therefore necessary to treat *Candida* with an antiyeast/antifungal, such as Nystatin, Diflucan, Mycostatin, etc., to control the toxins and take the pressure off the immune system. It is also beneficial to use supplements to improve the immune system. (See Appendix A—"Supplements for *Candida* and the Immune System.")

Gail Burton's Own *Candida* Story

I suffered for over 10 years with stomach pain, cramps, and bloating. I had been from doctor to doctor, but no one could help me. They just kept diagnosing me with spastic colon and prescribed more and more medications, which made me even worse.

I always thought I had something more than spastic colon. I even went to the University of California to see one of its head gastroenterologists, who did a colonoscopy on me. After the procedure, he said, "You have nothing more than spastic colon. I'll put you in the hospital and get you on an all bran diet, and that should take care of your problem." However, I felt I was too ill to try the diet, and thank goodness for that, because I was later found to be allergic to bran!

I remember a particularly warm day in California, in 1985. I loved being out-of-doors in that kind of weather. But I couldn't be outside, because I was so ill that I was bedridden. I had so much stomach pain and was so depressed; I actually felt I didn't want to live anymore. In those same devastating moments, the telephone rang. I had missed a nail appointment, and Justine, the manicurist, who had become my friend as well, knew I was very ill. She was calling to tell me about a doctor who could possibly help me. He was Dr. Michael Rosenbaum, an M.D., who specializes in Nutrition and Preventive Medicine. Just another doctor, I thought. Thank God I was wrong!

After examining me, Dr. Rosenbaum suspected that I had *Candida*, a word I had never heard before. He explained that we all have *Candida albicans* yeast in us, which lives harmlessly in our mucous membranes and other warm places in the body. However, antibiotics, steroids, stress, and other factors cause the yeast to become active and harmful. When he mentioned antibiotics, a bell went off in my head! My urologist had put me on Bactrim for a full year to prevent reoccurring urinary tract infections. I learned later that the antibacterial drug had wiped out most, if not all, of my good bacteria. Dr. Rosenbaum also suspected that I had low thyroid. "But my thyroid was tested just a couple of weeks ago, and it was normal," I protested. Dr. Rosenbaum insisted that he wanted to do special thyroid testing . . . a full-panel thyroid test.

The results of the full-panel thyroid test showed that my thyroid was so low that it was inflamed, and Dr. Rosenbaum prescribed medication for me. Thyroid dysfunction often goes hand-in-hand with *Candida*. *Candida* may cause the thyroid gland to malfunction or vice versa.

My *Candida* blood test results showed that I actually had chronic *Candidiasis*, and Dr. Rosenbaum immediately put me on the *Candida* Treatment Program. This consisted of the *Candida* Control Diet, Nystatin (an antiyeast/antifungal), with acidophilus and vitamin C to rebuild my immune system.

In the meantime, I attended one of Dr. Rosenbaum's *Candida* support group meetings and was surprised to discover that I was not the only one there who suffered from spastic colon, bloated stomach, poor memory, and extreme fatigue. I found out that those were typical *Candida* symptoms, as along with recurring headaches, hair loss, allergies, and many others.

The special *Candida* diet was difficult for me to stay on because it was so restrictive, but it did help my symptoms to improve. Therefore, I knew I had to stick with it. So I realized that the only way I could accomplish that was to have enjoyable recipes with good substitutions for problem ingredients. I did a great deal of experimentation with old recipes and created many new ones. As a result, I stayed on the diet. After six months, I was finally well.

Dr. Rosenbaum and his support group sampled many of my recipes and urged me to write a cookbook for other *Candida* sufferers. The rest is history, because *The Candida Control Cookbook* has been in publication since 1989, and is still going strong after several revisions and updates.

I am extremely grateful to Dr. Rosenbaum and the *Candida* Treatment Program that I can enjoy good health today.

VIII. Protecting Your Rights to Safe, Alternative Health Care

By Leo B. Cashman, Minneapolis Health Writer

It may be surprising to some of you when I say that your access to safe, alternative health care treatments is not assured.

While conventional medical treatment centers around prescription drugs, surgery, and radiation, more and more people are also seeking less-invasive, more-natural methods of treatment that involve changes in lifestyle and diet, as well as detoxification and avoidance of toxic exposures.

People want to understand the fundamental causes of illness, to bring about true healing. But those who offer the complementary and alternative forms of healing are vulnerable to being prosecuted, and consumer access to their health care services is correspondingly threatened.

We must seek to understand the nature of this problem. Then we must act together to change our state and federal laws, to protect our basic health freedoms.

Under the laws of most states, the definition of the practice of medicine is very broad. Anyone who seeks to help heal the pain, infirmity, or diseases of another person, or even to prevent illness, could be regarded as "practicing medicine." Unless such a person is exempted as a chiropractor, dentist, nurse or some other licensed practitioner, the person is violating the state's medical practice law.

So the homeopaths, herbalists, body workers, energy healers, and naturopaths, who in most states are unlicensed, can easily be charged with "the practice of medicine without a license."

There need not be any evidence of harm for such a prosecution to go forward.

The licensed practitioners who use complementary or alternative health care treatments may also be charged: The medical, dental, or other licensing board may charge them with practicing outside of the "standard of care."

There need not be any evidence of harm; support for the practitioner from his or her patients, from colleagues, or even from published scientific literature often carries no weight with the judge. The "standard of care" is written down nowhere, and basically turns out to be whatever the board's expert witness says it is. Thus, it turns out to be whatever the prevailing or conventional method of care is. So, licensure does not guarantee freedom from harassment; and being innovative and on the cutting edge of change, better than the usual care, can put a licensed practitioner into a legally vulnerable position.

Citizens for Health has led the response at the federal level, seeking to at least protect holistic M.D.s under the Access to Medical Treatment Act (AMTA). Consumers for Dental Choice (CDC) has organized a national campaign to protect mercury-free, holistic dentists from the attacks that they have faced in so many states.

In several states there have been legal reforms to protect the various kinds of practitioners; a group called the Minnesota Natural Health Coalition Action Network has organized to protect the whole gamut of alternative health practitioners, both licensed and unlicensed, in one innovative piece of legislation.

As an action group, they have also organized to support the election of candidates who support their reforms and have educated not only legislators, but also the governor and attorney general about their concerns. Involvement of a large number of citizens should carry the day on these legal reform issues. I urge you to find out what is happening on the health freedom front in your state, and join in.

If we all join together, we can pass the needed reforms and assure our access to the kind of excellent, innovative health care we need.

Resources

Two national umbrella organizations for the health freedom movement can put you in touch with health freedom groups in your state:

National Health Freedom Coalition (educational nonprofit)
National Health Freedom Action (nonprofit that lobbies for health freedom)

NOTE: Both organizations above can be contacted at:
Address: 2136 Ford Pkwy, Box 218, St Paul, MN 55116
Phone: 651-690-0732

IX. How to Start a *Candida* Support Group

If you don't have a *Candida* support group in your area, it is easy to start one. Begin by selecting a date and a place for a meeting, such as your house or apartment. If you live in an apartment complex, perhaps there is a recreation center where you can meet. Next, make flyers, with wording similar to the following:

Do you suffer from *Candida*, yeast infection?

(You could also add Lupus, Fibromyalgia,
Chronic Fatigue Syndrome, etc.)

Come to a *Candida* Support Group Meeting.

Time:_____ Date: _____ Place: _____

Put the flyers up at all of the health and natural foods stores, and co-ops in your area. Include an email address for people to contact you.

It's also a good idea to deliver or mail flyers to offices of health care professionals who are knowledgeable about *Candida* and who treat the condition. Many of those doctors could be holistic or natural health care professionals. You also might ask them if they would be willing to speak on *Candida* and related conditions at one of your meetings.

When your group is larger, contact a church, county recreation center, or library to arrange for a meeting place. Your group would be a nonprofit organization, so there will probably be no charge at any of those locations.

You could start out with just a few people and end up with many, as I did. My *Candida* support group started out with just five people; we met in my home. However, when the group grew, we met at a library in Burlingame, California. We ended up with about 100 members. Also, after I moved to Minnesota, Dr. Keith Sehnert urged me to start the Twin Cities *Candida* Support Group, which I did. We met at a library in Edina, Minnesota, where the group grew to 150 members. Both libraries supplied my meetings with microphones, movie projectors, VCRs, TVs, slide screens, and tables, whenever I requested them. You should also request these or any other items you need.

Also, it's a good idea to take out books from the library that deal with *Candida* or related conditions and have them on hand to recommend to the members

In addition to having health care professionals speak at the meetings, I asked recovered members to speak to the group about how they got well. Sometimes there would be a member who wanted to speak about a particular product or products that helped in their recovery. The products and any informational material pertaining to *Candida* and related conditions were displayed on a table at the meetings.

When the group got larger, I organized a committee to help phone and remind members of meetings and programs. However, when the membership became too much for them to handle, mailings were sent out instead. Then, at those meetings, a basket was passed around for donations to help cover the cost of printing and mailing. Be sure and get everyone's email address.

I felt it was extremely important to try to promote a positive attitude in my members. Rather than their focusing on the negative aspects of their conditions, I encouraged them to concentrate on any progress they had made. It would be beneficial for you to do the same.

Also, there were many members who didn't get the support they needed from families and friends. Therefore, support group meetings were very important to them, because they enabled them to not feel so alone in their struggles to recover.

One of the most important things I learned from my members is that they wanted to have a special period during the meetings when they could be a real support group. To accomplish this, they wanted to form a circle with their chairs, and just sit and talk to other members about experiences with *Candida* and related conditions. I found this to be extremely beneficial for their healing process. I am certain that if you allot time for this special process, you also will find it to be very helpful.

Appendix A
Supplements for *Candida* and the Immune System

Please note that most of the products in this section can be found in or may be ordered through your health or natural foods store, or co-op, unless otherwise indicated.

Acidophilus (available in capsules or powder) has been found to be a good immune builder, because it is capable of replacing the good bacteria that the body may be lacking.

Aqua Flora has been known to be one of the many treatments for yeast infection. It is a water-based homeopathic remedy with three phases. Website: www.aqua-flora.net e-mail: info@aqua-flora.net; phone: 1-888-452-4968

Bifidus (also available in some acidophilus products) has been found to be beneficial for the intestines.

Capricin™ (available in pills or capsules) contains caprylic acid, which is known as a nutritional broad spectrum fungicide for *Candida*. Also, it has been found to help restore and maintain the balance of yeast, bacteria, and other microorganisms in the colon.

Charcoal (available in tablets and capsules) has been found to aid diarrhea, bloating, and gas.

Chromium Picolinate™ has been known to help cravings and stabilize hypoglycemia (low blood sugar), a condition often associated with *Candida*.

Coenzyme Q10 (CoQ10) has been known to enhance immune system cell performance.

Echinacea is an antioxidant and also known to be a good immune system builder.

Ester-C® has been known to help support the immune system. It has also been found to be more beneficial than regular vitamin C, because it is coated to prevent upsetting the digestive tract and can be easily absorbed. By Natrol. Website: www.natrol.com

Garlic, odorless. Many of the antiyeast/antifungal properties are lost from fresh garlic after it is cooked, while odorless garlic pills or capsules contain most of them.

Grapefruit extract (*Citrus Paradisi*) is known to be a good antiyeast/antifungal and has also been found to be helpful in eliminating parasites.

Hydrochloric acid (available in capsules or tablets) is a digestive aid that replaces gastric juices, which may be lacking in the digestive system. *Caution: Hydrochloric acid in liquid form is not recommended because it could possibly damage tooth enamel.*

Pau D'Arco (available in capsules and tinctures) has been known to be a good antiyeast/antifungal.

Peroxide has been known to be helpful in eliminating thrush (a white-coated tongue), which is *Candida*, as well as other mouth infections. Mix with water for a mouthwash.

Pine bark is an antioxidant and known to be a good immune system builder.

Taheebo Tea (*also known as Pau D'Arco, La pacho, Ipe Roxo, Tabeuia, Tecoma, Bow Stick*). This tea from the bark of trees grown in the rain forests of South America, is free of fungus and is a natural antiyeast/antifungal for *Candida* and CRC treatment. Also, once steeped and cooled, the tea can be made into compresses for skin rashes.

Vitamin C (available in capsules, liquid, or tablets) has been found to enhance the immune system and protects against damage by toxins from *Candida albicans. Caution: Regular*

Vitamin C is ascorbic acid and can upset the digestive system. (See Ester-C® above.)

Zinc (available in tablets) has been found to be beneficial for internal healing.

Zinc oxide ointment has been found to promote skin healing.

Appendix B
Resources

Mark A. Breiner, DDS
  www.wholebodydentistry.com
  1-203-799-6353
Gail Burton's website:
  www.immunefix.com;
  E-mail: gburton@immunefix.com
Candida-Candidaisis Homepage:
  www.curezone.com/diseases/candida
The Candida Page:
  www.candidapage.com
Candida-Yeast, by Wm. G. Crook, M.D.:
  http://candida-yeast.com
The Candida Yeast Answer,
  by Gary Carlsen, R.H., Director, Candida Wellness Center:
  www.internet-promotion.com/ candida/yeast/infections/
Bruce R. MacFarland, Ph.D., CCN;
  The *Candida* Program.
  www.candidaprogram.com
Michael McNett, M.D., director of Paragon Clinic, specializing
  in *Candida,* fibromyalgia, and myofascial pain syndrome.
  www.paragonclinic.com
  E-mail: mmcnett@paragonclinic.com;
  Phone: 773-604-5321
  Address: 4332 N. Elston Ave., Chicago, IL 60641
Michael E. Rosenbaum, M.D. Phone: 415-927-9450;
  Fax: 927-2596; www.michaelrosenbaummd.com;
  E-mail:mermd@michaelrosenbaummd.com
  Address: 300 Tamal Plaza, Suite 120,
  Corte Madera, CA, 94925.

National *Candida* Society:
    www.candida-society.org.uk
Project Inform; oral *Candidiasis* (Thrush):
    www.projinf.org/fs/candida.html

Appendix C
Recommended Readings

Candida: A Twentieth Century Disease, by Shirley S. Lorenzani, Ph.D. (Keats Publishing, 1986)

Candida-Related Complex: What Your Doctor Might Be Missing, by Christine Winderlin with Keith Sehnert, M.D. (Taylor Publishing Co., 1996)

Conquering Yeast Infections: The Non-Drug Solution, by S. Colet Lahoz, RN, MS, LAc (Pentland Press, Inc., 1996)

The Cure for All Cancers, by Hulda Regehr Clark, Ph.D., N.D. (New Century Press, 1993)

The Cure for All Diseases, by Hulda Regehr Clark, (ProMotion Publishing, 1995)

The Garden Within: Acidophilus-Candida Connection, by Keith W. Sehnert, M.D. (Health World Inc., 1989)

Guess What Came to Dinner: Parasites and Your Health, by Ann Louise Gittleman (Avery Publishers Group, 1993)

I'm Sorry, but Your Perfume Makes Me Sick: and So Does Almost Everything Else that Smells, by Kathy Glenn (Bluebird Books, Carlisle Print, 1997)

Love, Medicine and Miracles; Lessons Learned about Self-Healing from a Surgeon's Experience with Exceptional Patients, by Bernie S. Siegel, M.D., (Harper Perennial, 1990, 1986)

The Missing Diagnosis, by C. Orian Truss (Box 26508, Birmingham, AL 35226, 1983-1986)

Solving the Puzzle of Chronic Fatigue Syndrome, by Michael Rosenbaum, M.D. and Murray Susser, M.D. (Life Sciences Press, 1992)

Whole-Body Dentistry: Discover the Missing Piece to Better Health, by Mark A. Breiner, DDS (Quantum Health Press, LLC, 1999)

Wilson's Syndrome: The Miracle of Feeling Well, by E. Denis Wilson, M.D. (Wilson Syndrome Foundation, P.O. Box 539, Summerfield, FL 34492, phone: 800-621-7006, website: www.wilsonssyndrome.com)

The Whole Way to Allergy Relief & Prevention: A Doctor's Complete Guide to Treatment and Self-Care, by Jacqueline Krohn (Hartley & Marks, 1996)

The Yeast Connection, by Wm. Crook, M.D. (Professional Books, 1983)

The Yeast Connection and the Woman, by Wm. Crook, M.D. (Professional Books, 1995)

The Yeast Syndrome, by John Parks Trowbridge, M.D. and Morton Walker, D/P.M. (Bantam Books, 1986)

Your Body Believes Every Word You Say: The Language of the Body/Mind Connection, by Barbara Hoberman Levine (WordsWork Press, 2000)

Index

A Helpful 14-Day Journal

The following pages are a daily journal for you to use for 14 days. It is important that you start recording in this journal as soon as possible.

The journal is a self-help tool, because it will enable you to monitor the foods you are eating, the medications, supplements and remedies you may be taking and what symptoms you may be experiencing.

It is important to record the foods you eat, because you will be able to see if you are consuming too many sweets and complex carbohydrates, upon which the *Candida albicans* yeast thrive. Also, many times you may eat the same food too often; less than four days apart. As a result, you may develop an allergy to it. This is because you may have a sensitive digestive system, which is typical of people who have *Candida.*

In addition, if you are taking any *Candida* medication or natural products, you may be taking more than you should. It has been found that many times *Candida* sufferers are so desperate to get well that they take more than one and sometimes several remedies at a time, which actually complicates their recovery.

Furthermore, when you record your symptoms, you will be able to keep good track of them and possibly what precipitates them. *Candida* sufferers can have many symptoms from head to toe. The most common ones are listed in Chapter III—Self-Help *Candida* Evaluations: Do You Have *Candida*-Related Symptoms?

It is also important to record your thoughts and feelings. Depression is a common symptom of *Candida,* as well as anxiety.

At the end of the journal you will find a self-evaluation page, intended for you to personally review your progress.

I wish you the best of luck as you begin your journey on the road to recovery.

Gail Burton

DAY 1

BREAKFAST:

SNACK:

LUNCH:

SNACK:

DINNER:

SNACK:

MEDICATIONS:

SUPPLEMENTS:

CANDIDA REMEDIES, IF ANY:

SYMPTOMS:

THOUGHTS/FEELINGS:

DAY 2

BREAKFAST:

SNACK:

LUNCH:

SNACK:

DINNER:

SNACK:

MEDICATIONS:

SUPPLEMENTS:

CANDIDA REMEDIES, IF ANY:

SYMPTOMS:

THOUGHTS/FEELINGS:

DAY 3

BREAKFAST:

SNACK:

LUNCH:

SNACK:

DINNER:

SNACK:

MEDICATIONS:

SUPPLEMENTS:

CANDIDA REMEDIES, IF ANY:

SYMPTOMS:

THOUGHTS/FEELINGS:

DAY 4

BREAKFAST:

SNACK:

LUNCH:

SNACK:

DINNER:

SNACK:

MEDICATIONS:

SUPPLEMENTS:

CANDIDA REMEDIES, IF ANY:

SYMPTOMS:

THOUGHTS/FEELINGS:

DAY 5

BREAKFAST:

SNACK:

LUNCH:

SNACK:

DINNER:

SNACK:

MEDICATIONS:

SUPPLEMENTS:

CANDIDA REMEDIES, IF ANY:

SYMPTOMS:

THOUGHTS/FEELINGS:

DAY 6

BREAKFAST:

SNACK:

LUNCH:

SNACK:

DINNER:

SNACK:

MEDICATIONS:

SUPPLEMENTS:

CANDIDA REMEDIES, IF ANY:

SYMPTOMS:

THOUGHTS/FEELINGS:

DAY 7

BREAKFAST:

SNACK:

LUNCH:

SNACK:

DINNER:

SNACK:

MEDICATIONS:

SUPPLEMENTS:

CANDIDA REMEDIES, IF ANY:

SYMPTOMS:

THOUGHTS/FEELINGS:

DAY 8

BREAKFAST:

SNACK:

LUNCH:

SNACK:

DINNER:

SNACK:

MEDICATIONS:

SUPPLEMENTS:

CANDIDA REMEDIES, IF ANY:

SYMPTOMS:

THOUGHTS/FEELINGS:

DAY 9

BREAKFAST:

SNACK:

LUNCH:

SNACK:

DINNER:

SNACK:

MEDICATIONS:

SUPPLEMENTS:

CANDIDA REMEDIES, IF ANY:

SYMPTOMS:

THOUGHTS/FEELINGS:

DAY 10

BREAKFAST:

SNACK:

LUNCH:

SNACK:

DINNER:

SNACK:

MEDICATIONS:

SUPPLEMENTS:

CANDIDA REMEDIES, IF ANY:

SYMPTOMS:

THOUGHTS/FEELINGS:

DAY 11

BREAKFAST:

SNACK:

LUNCH:

SNACK:

DINNER:

SNACK:

MEDICATIONS:

SUPPLEMENTS:

CANDIDA REMEDIES, IF ANY:

SYMPTOMS:

THOUGHTS/FEELINGS:

DAY 12

BREAKFAST:

SNACK:

LUNCH:

SNACK:

DINNER:

SNACK:

MEDICATIONS:

SUPPLEMENTS:

CANDIDA REMEDIES, IF ANY:

SYMPTOMS:

THOUGHTS/FEELINGS:

DAY 13

BREAKFAST:

SNACK:

LUNCH:

SNACK:

DINNER:

SNACK:

MEDICATIONS:

SUPPLEMENTS:

CANDIDA REMEDIES, IF ANY:

SYMPTOMS:

THOUGHTS/FEELINGS:

DAY 14

BREAKFAST:

SNACK:

LUNCH:

SNACK:

DINNER:

SNACK:

MEDICATIONS:

SUPPLEMENTS:

CANDIDA REMEDIES, IF ANY:

SYMPTOMS:

THOUGHTS/FEELINGS:

Self-Evaluation of My 14-Day Journal

Please answer the following questions after reviewing your 14-day journal:

1. Did I have a large amount of sugars and complex carbohydrates?

2. Did I take too many medications?

3. Did I take too many supplements?

4. If I had *Candida* therapy, did I use more than one remedy at a time?

5. Have my symptoms improved?

6. Has my thinking or feelings changed?

7. What steps do I need to take in order to improve my health?

Titles Published by Aslan

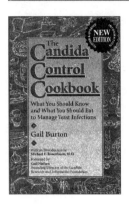

The Candida Control Cookbook What You Should Know And What You Should Eat To Manage Yeast Infections
by Gail Burton
$14.95
ISBN 0-944031-67-6

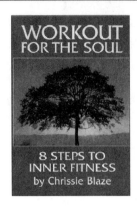

Workout for the Soul: 8 Steps to Inner Fitness
by Chrissie Blaze
$14.95
ISBN 0-944031-90-0

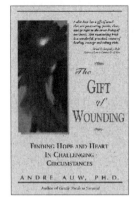

The Gift of Wounding: Finding Hope & Heart in Challenging Circumstances
by Andre Auw Ph.D.
$13.95
ISBN 0-944031-79-X

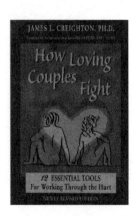

How Loving Couples Fight: 12 Essential Tools for Working Through the Hurt
by James L Creighton Ph.D.
$16.95
ISBN 0-944031-71-4

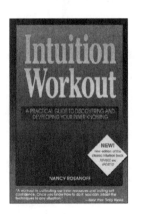

Intuition Workout: A Practical Guide To Discovering & Developing Your Inner Knowing
by Nancy Rosanoff
$12.95
ISBN 0-944031-14-5

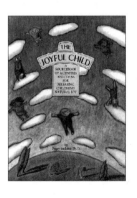

The Joyful Child: A Sourcebook of Activities and Ideas for Releasing Children's Natural Joy
by Peggy Jenkins Ph.D.
$16.95
ISBN 0-944031-66-8

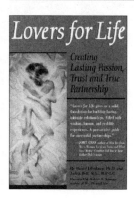

*Lovers For Life: Creating
Lasting Passion, Trust
and True Partnership*
by Daniel Ellenberg Ph.D.
& Judith Bell M.S., MFCC
$16.95
ISBN 0-944031-61-7

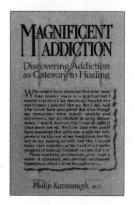

*Magnificent Addiction:
Discovering Addiction as
Gateway to Healing*
by Philip R. Kavanaugh, M.D.
$14.95
ISBN 0-944031-36-6

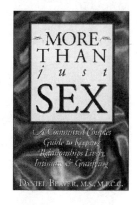

*More Than Just Sex:
A Committed Couples
Guide to Keeping
Relationships Lively,
Intimate & Gratifying*
by Daniel Beaver M.S., MFCC
$12.95
ISBN0-944031-35-8

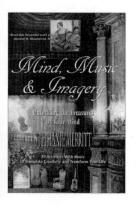

*Mind, Music & Imagery:
Unlocking the Treasures
of Your Mind*
by Stephanie Merritt
$13.95
ISBN 0-944031-62-5

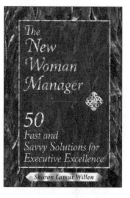

*New Woman Manager: 50
Fast & Savvy Solutions for
Executive Excellence*
by Sharon Lamhut Willen
$14.95
ISBN 0-944031-11-0

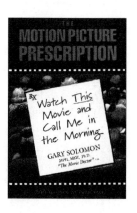

*The Motion Picture
Pre-scription Watch This
Movie and Call Me in The
Morning: 200 Movies to help
you heal life's problems*
by Gary Solomon Ph.D.
"The Movie Doctor"
$12.95
ISBN 0-944031-27-7

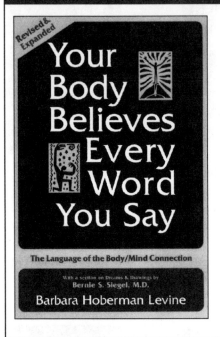
Sing and Change the World
By David Edward Dayton, $16.95; ISBN 0-944031-92-7

The Sacred Weave
By Marianne Franzese Chasen, $13.95; ISBN 0-944031-91-9

To order any of Aslan's titles send a check or money order for the price of the book plus Shipping & Handling
> **Book Rate** $3 for 1st book.; $1.00 for each additional book
> **First Class** $4 for 1st book; $1.50 for each additional book

Send to: **Aslan Publishing**
2490 Black Rock Turnpike # 342
Fairfield CT 06825

To receive a current catalog: please call (800) 786–5427 or (203) 372–0300
E-mail us at: **info@aslanpublishing.com**
Visit our website at **www.aslanpublishing.com**

Our authors are available for seminars, workshops, and lectures. For further information or to reach a specific author, please call or email Aslan Publishing.